SUPER EASY
IC DIET COOKBOOK

1500 Days of Nourishing Recipes for a Healthy Bladder

HARRIET BARRET, MS, RDN

Copyright © 2025 by.Harriet Barret, MS, RDN. All rights reserved.

No part of this publication may be reproduced, distributed, or transmitted in any form or by any means, including photocopying, recording, or other electronic or mechanical methods, without the prior written permission of the publisher, except in the case of brief quotations embodied in critical reviews and other noncommercial uses permitted by copyright law.

Legal Notice:
This book is protected by copyright law and is intended for personal use only. Without explicit permission from the publisher or author, you are prohibited from altering, distributing, selling, quoting, or paraphrasing any part of the content.

Disclaimer:

The recipes and information in The SUper Easy IC Diet Cookbook are provided for educational and informational purposes only. They are not meant to replace professional medical advice, diagnosis, or treatment. Always consult your physician or another qualified healthcare provider if you have any concerns about your health or medical conditions. The author and publisher are not responsible for any negative effects or outcomes that may result from using the information or recipes provided. Please prioritize the advice of your healthcare professional when making dietary or health-related decisions.

Table of Contents

Introduction..................................13
Understanding Interstitial Cystitis (IC)..................................14
The Role of Diet in Managing IC..................................16
Core Principles of the IC Diet   17
How This Cookbook Can Benefit You..................................18
Tips for Successfully Adhering to the IC Diet..................................19
Identifying Trigger Foods and Safe Alternatives..................................20
Bladder-Friendly Alternatives   21

Chapter 1: Breakfasts to Start Your Day Right..................................24
Oatmeal with Blueberries & Almond Milk..................................25
Quinoa Breakfast Bowl with Banana & Chia Seeds..................................27

Whole Wheat Pancakes with Maple Syrup..................................29
Scrambled Eggs with Spinach & Mushrooms..............................31
Coconut Yogurt Parfait with Strawberries................................33
Avocado Toast on Gluten-Free Bread...35
Rice Pudding with Cinnamon and Honey....................................37
Banana Nut Smoothie 39
Sweet Potato Hash 41
Apple Cinnamon Quinoa....................43

Chapter 2: Nutritious Salads & Light Meals..................................45
Spinach & Chicken Salad with Olive Oil Vinaigrette............................46
Grilled Salmon Salad with Avocado 48
Carrot & Cucumber Ribbon Salad 50
Roasted Beetroot Salad with Arugula...................................52
Quinoa & Veggie Power Salad 54

Chopped Cabbage Salad with Lemon Dressing..................56
Turkey & Cranberry Spinach Salad   58
Roasted Sweet Potato & Kale Salad   60
Simple Avocado & Tomato Salad   62
Zucchini Noodles with Lemon   64

Chapter 3: Hearty Soups & Stews..................66
Creamy Carrot & Ginger Soup   67
Chicken & Vegetable Broth   69
Butternut Squash Soup with Coconut Milk..................71
Potato Leek Soup   73
Lentil & Spinach Stew   75
Sweet Potato & Red Lentil Soup   77
Tomato Basil Soup   80
Broccoli & Cauliflower Cream Soup..................82
Beef & Root Vegetable Stew   84
Chicken Bone Broth with Carrots   86

Chapter 4: Main Dishes for Lunch & Dinner..................88
Grilled Lemon Herb Chicken with Rice..................89
Baked Salmon with Steamed Veggies..................91
Veggie-Stuffed Bell Peppers   95
Zucchini Noodles with Chicken & Olive Oil..................95
Turkey Meatballs with Quinoa   97
Grilled Cod with Sweet Potato Mash..................99
Eggplant Parmesan   103
Roasted Chicken with Green Beans..................105
Baked Tilapia with Sautéed Spinach..................107
Quinoa & Vegetable Stir-Fry   109

Chapter 5: Sides & Vegetables..............111
Roasted Garlic & Herb Sweet Potatoes..............112
Steamed Asparagus with Lemon Zest..............114
Sautéed Spinach with Olive Oil & Garlic..............116
Baked Zucchini Fries 118
Cauliflower Rice Pilaf 120
Mashed Butternut Squash 122
Roasted Brussels Sprouts with Apple Cider Vinegar..............124
Sautéed Green Beans with Almonds..............126
Carrot & Cucumber Sticks with Hummus..............128
Grilled Veggie Skewers 130

Chapter 6: Healthy Snacks & Treats..................132
Turmeric and Ginger Tea — 133
Apple Slices with Peanut Butter — 135
Rice Cakes with Avocado Spread — 137
Cucumber & Cream Cheese Bites..................139
Carrot Sticks with Tzatziki — 141
Baked Zucchini Chips — 142
Homemade Popcorn with Olive Oil..................144
Frozen Yogurt Bark with Berries — 146
Coconut Macaroons with Fruit Popsicles..................148
Almond Protein Bars — 150

Chapter 7: Smoothies & Refreshing Beverages..................152
Green Smoothie with Spinach & Banana..................153
Berry Almond Milk Smoothie — 155
Tropical Mango Coconut Smoothie — 157
Cucumber & Mint Infused Water.......159

Sweet Carrot & Apple Juice.................161
Pear & Ginger Smoothie....................163
Lemon & Honey Detox Drink   165
Blueberry Yogurt Smoothie................167
Avocado & Peach Smoothie   169
Cantaloupe & Lime Slush..................171

Chapter 8: wholesome Desserts..173
Coconut Rice Pudding   174
Vanilla Almond Cake   176
Blueberry Sorbet..............................178
Banana Ice Cream.............................180
Lemon Curd Cups.............................182
Chocolate Avocado Mousse   184
Pear & Cinnamon Crisp   186
Baked Apple with Almond Butter   188
Carrot Cake......................................190
Chia Pudding with Berries................192

Chapter 9: Meal Planning & Prep Tips..................................194
How to Plan Your IC-Friendly 30-Day Meal Plan..................................195
Batch Cooking and Freezer-Friendly Recipes..................................210
Grocery Shopping on the IC Diet   210
Best Pantry Staples for IC Diet Success..................................210

Conclusion..................................212
Final Thoughts on Maintaining Long-Term Bladder Health..................212
Monitoring Your Progress   213
Support and Community Resources for IC..................................213
..................................214

DEDICATION

This book is dedicated to every person living with Interstitial Cystitis (IC), who battles through pain and uncertainty every single day. I see you, and I feel the weight of what you're enduring—the sleepless nights, the constant discomfort, and the frustration of not being understood. The invisible nature of IC can make your journey incredibly isolating, but through your resilience, strength, and unwavering courage, you continue to fight. This book is a tribute to your spirit and a reminder that you are not alone.

I also want to acknowledge the love and support of family, friends, and medical practitioners who have been there every step of the way. To the nutritionists, doctors, and caregivers whose guidance, knowledge, and compassion make all the difference—thank you. Your tireless efforts to improve lives and offer hope have been instrumental in making this cookbook come to life. Your belief in the power of healing, and your willingness to walk alongside those living with IC, inspire me every day.

May this book be a small beacon of hope, a source of comfort, and a reminder that with every challenge, there is strength, and with every step forward, healing is possible.

INTRODUCTION

Hello, and welcome! I'm Harriet Barret, and I'm thrilled to present this cookbook to you. I've carefully curated this collection of recipes with the intention of not only delighting your taste buds but also promoting your overall well-being. If you're living with Interstitial Cystitis (IC), you understand how challenging it can be, but I truly believe that the right food choices can make a significant difference in how you feel and help nourish your body in a healing way. These recipes are designed to support you on your journey toward better health, bringing comfort, balance, and relief, all through nourishing and delicious meals.

Understanding Interstitial Cystitis (IC)

Interstitial Cystitis (IC), also known as Bladder Pain Syndrome (BPS), is a long-term condition that results in bladder and pelvic discomfort. It is frequently associated with a strong urge to urinate. Although IC can affect anyone, it is more prevalent in women. The precise cause of IC is not fully understood, but it is believed to involve a mix of factors such as bladder inflammation, a damaged bladder lining, and nerve dysfunction.

Types of Interstitial Cystitis:

1. Non-ulcerative IC: This is the more common form and is characterized by the absence of visible ulcers in the bladder. While inflammation may vary, there is no noticeable ulceration in the bladder lining.

2. Ulcerative IC (Hunner's Ulcers): This rarer type involves visible sores or ulcers on the bladder wall. These ulcers can result in more intense pain and discomfort.

Causes of Interstitial Cystitis:

Although the exact cause remains unclear, several factors are thought to contribute to the development of IC:

Bladder Lining Damage: The bladder's protective lining may become weakened, allowing irritants to penetrate the bladder wall.

Autoimmune Response: The immune system may mistakenly attack bladder tissue, leading to inflammation.

Nerve Issues: In some cases, nerve signaling becomes abnormal, increasing bladder sensitivity.

Genetics: A family history and genetic predisposition can play a role in the development of IC.

Symptoms of Interstitial Cystitis:
- Persistent pelvic pain or bladder discomfort
- Frequent urination, especially at night
- An urgent need to urinate
- Painful urination
- Discomfort during intercourse
- Pressure or discomfort in the lower abdomen
- Flare-ups that worsen with stress, certain foods, or other triggers

The Role of Diet in Managing IC:
Diet is a critical aspect of managing IC. Certain foods may irritate the bladder and exacerbate symptoms, while others can help alleviate

inflammation. An IC-friendly diet focuses on avoiding bladder irritants and incorporating foods that promote bladder health.

The IC Diet: An Overview

The IC diet is designed to eliminate foods and drinks that are known to irritate the bladder. It encourages an anti-inflammatory, balanced approach to eating, focusing on foods that are gentle on the bladder while providing essential nutrients.

Core Principles of the IC Diet:

1. Avoiding Acidic and Irritating Foods: Many people with IC find relief by cutting out foods and drinks that are acidic or overly spicy. Common triggers include citrus fruits, tomatoes, coffee, and alcohol.

2. Incorporating Alkaline, Bladder-Friendly Foods: The IC diet focuses on foods that help maintain a neutral or alkaline body pH, such as bananas, pears, oatmeal, and select vegetables.

3. Maintaining Proper Hydration: It's important to stay hydrated by drinking plenty of water throughout the day and avoiding excessive caffeine or alcohol, both of which can irritate the bladder.

How This Cookbook Can Benefit You

This IC-friendly cookbook is designed to assist those with Interstitial Cystitis by providing easy-to-follow recipes that are free from common bladder irritants. The cookbook features a wide range of meal options meant to support bladder health, such as:

- Breakfast dishes like oatmeal and smoothies that are gentle on the bladder.
- Lunch and dinner recipes with lean proteins, vegetables, and whole grains.
- Snack suggestions that avoid common IC triggers, such as mild fruits and rice cakes.

By preparing these recipes, you can enjoy nutritious meals without worrying about aggravating your bladder.

Tips for Successfully Adhering to the IC Diet

Staying on track with an IC-friendly diet can be difficult, especially when eating out or in social situations. Here are some helpful tips for successfully following the IC diet:

1. Plan Meals in Advance: Preparing meals and snacks ahead of time ensures you stay on course and avoid accidental consumption of irritants.

2. Track Your Food: Keep a food diary to monitor what you eat and how it affects your symptoms. This can help you identify personal triggers.

3. Examine Food Labels: Processed foods may contain hidden irritants like artificial sweeteners or preservatives. Always check the labels of packaged foods before buying.

4. Cook Your Own Meals: Preparing your own meals offers control over the ingredients, ensuring that they're safe for your bladder.

5. Be Aware of Common Triggers: Although triggers vary by person, foods like spicy dishes, caffeine, alcohol, citrus fruits, tomatoes, and artificial sweeteners are often problematic for people with IC.

Identifying Trigger Foods and Safe Alternatives

Certain trigger foods can significantly aggravate IC symptoms, but there are many safe alternatives that are bladder-friendly.

Foods to Avoid:

1. Citrus fruits: Such as oranges, lemons, limes, and grapefruits.

2. Tomatoes: Including sauces, salsas, and ketchup.

3. Caffeinated Beverages: Coffee, tea, and energy drinks.
4. Alcohol: Particularly beer, wine, and spirits.
5. Artificial Sweeteners: Such as aspartame and sucralose.
6. Spicy Dishes: Hot peppers and dishes with chili or curry.
7. Carbonated Drinks: Soda and sparkling water.

Bladder-Friendly Alternatives:

Fruits: Pears, apples (peeled), blueberries, and melons.
Vegetables: Carrots, zucchini, leafy greens, and broccoli.
Grain: Oats, quinoa, and rice.
Lean Proteins: Chicken, turkey, and fish (grilled or baked, not fried).
Herbal Teas: Chamomile, peppermint, and ginger tea (without caffeine).

Cooking for a Healthy Bladder: A Practical Guide

When preparing meals for IC, it's crucial to choose ingredients that are both bladder-friendly and nutritious. Here are some general guidelines to follow:

1. Prioritize Fresh Ingredients: Fresh fruits, vegetables, and proteins are always the safest choice. Canned goods can contain preservatives and added acids that irritate the bladder.
2. Use Mild Herbs and Spices: Instead of hot spices, try using basil, oregano, thyme, and parsley to add flavor without irritation.
3. Minimize Processed Foods: Processed foods are often high in salt, preservatives, and additives that may irritate the bladder.
4. Healthy Fats: Olive oil, avocado, and coconut oil are excellent sources of healthy fats and should be used in moderation during cooking.

5. Incorporate Anti-inflammatory Foods: Ingredients like turmeric, ginger, and flaxseeds help reduce inflammation and can be beneficial for managing IC.

By following these cooking guidelines and incorporating bladder-friendly recipes, you can enjoy a variety of meals that support overall health and well-being.

Managing Interstitial Cystitis (IC) involves understanding how diet affects bladder health. By adopting an IC-friendly diet, avoiding common trigger foods, and including nourishing ingredients in your meals, you can minimize symptoms and enhance your quality of life. This cookbook offers a collection of bladder-friendly meals that can help you along your journey to better health. Always remember to consult with a healthcare professional before making significant changes to your diet.

Chapter 1

Breakfasts to Start Your Day Right

In this chapter, we'll explore breakfast recipes tailored for an IC (Interstitial Cystitis) diet, designed to nourish and energize you while supporting bladder health. A well-chosen breakfast sets the stage for the day, offering essential nutrients without irritating ingredients. We'll show you how to pick the right ingredients, prepare meals, and customize them for your specific needs. Let's kickstart your mornings with delicious, bladder-friendly breakfasts!

1. Oatmeal with Blueberries & Almond Milk

Preparation Time:
- 10 minutes
- Serves: 2

Ingredients:
- 1 cup rolled oats
- 2 cups unsweetened almond milk
- 1/2 cup fresh blueberries
- 1 tablespoon chia seeds (optional)
- A pinch of cinnamon (optional)

Instructions:
1. In a medium saucepan, bring almond milk to a simmer over medium heat.
2. Add oats to the simmering almond milk and stir occasionally, cooking for about 5-7 minutes, or until the oats are soft and the mixture thickens.

3. Once the oatmeal is ready, remove it from the heat and top with fresh blueberries, chia seeds, and a sprinkle of cinnamon.
4. Serve warm for a cozy, comforting breakfast.

Nutritional Value (per serving):
- Calories: 180
- Protein: 6g
- Fat: 7g
- Carbs: 27g
- Fiber: 6g
- Sugars: 7g

Tips:
- Make sure to choose unsweetened almond milk to avoid excess sugar.
- You can substitute the blueberries with strawberries or apples, depending on what works best for your needs.

2. Quinoa Breakfast Bowl with Banana & Chia Seeds

Preparation Time:
- 10 minutes
- Serves: 2

Ingredients:
- 1 cup cooked quinoa (cooled)
- 1 ripe banana, sliced
- 1 tablespoon chia seeds
- 1 tablespoon honey (optional)
- A pinch of cinnamon (optional)
- 1/2 cup unsweetened almond milk

Instructions:
1. Cook the quinoa according to package directions, then allow it to cool slightly.
2. In a bowl, combine the quinoa with almond milk to give it a creamy consistency.
3. Top with sliced banana, chia seeds, a drizzle of honey (if desired), and a sprinkle of cinnamon.
4. Stir to combine, and serve.

Nutritional Value (per serving):
- Calories: 250
- Protein: 6g
- Fat: 6g
- Carbs: 42g
- Fiber: 6g
- Sugars: 12g

Tips:
- If you find bananas too strong for your digestive needs, consider replacing them with blueberries or a handful of papaya.
- Quinoa is a naturally gluten-free grain, making it a suitable alternative for those sensitive to certain grains.

3. Whole Wheat Pancakes with Maple Syrup

Preparation Time:
- 15 minutes
- Serves: 2

Ingredients:
- 1 cup whole wheat flour
- 1 teaspoon baking powder
- 1/4 teaspoon salt
- 1 cup unsweetened almond milk
- 1 egg
- 1 teaspoon vanilla extract
- 1 tablespoon olive oil or coconut oil
- Maple syrup (for serving)

Instructions:
1. In a bowl, whisk together whole wheat flour, baking powder, and salt.
2. In another bowl, combine almond milk, egg, vanilla extract, and olive oil. Pour the wet

ingredients into the dry ingredients and mix until just combined.

3. Heat a non-stick skillet over medium heat and lightly grease with a bit of coconut oil.

4. Pour small amounts of batter onto the skillet to form pancakes. Cook each pancake for 2-3 minutes on each side until golden brown.

5. Serve warm with a drizzle of maple syrup.

Nutritional Value (per serving):
- Calories: 220
- Protein: 6g
- Fat: 7g
- Carbs: 32g
- Fiber: 4g
- Sugars: 9g

Tips:
- Whole wheat flour is high in fiber, but if it's too harsh, consider using oat flour for a gentler alternative.

- Maple syrup can be used sparingly to avoid excess sweetness and to ensure it complements the meal.

4. Scrambled Eggs with Spinach & Mushrooms

Preparation Time:
- 10 minutes
- Serves: 2

Ingredients:
- 4 large eggs
- 1/2 cup fresh spinach, chopped
- 1/2 cup mushrooms, sliced
- 1 tablespoon olive oil or coconut oil
- Salt and pepper to taste (optional)

Instructions:

1. Heat olive oil in a pan over medium heat. Add the sliced mushrooms and cook for about 2 minutes, until soft.
2. Add the spinach to the pan and cook for another minute until wilted.
3. Crack the eggs into a bowl, whisk, and pour over the veggies. Stir gently, cooking until the eggs are fully scrambled and cooked through.
4. Serve immediately.

Nutritional Value (per serving):

- Calories: 220
- Protein: 14g
- Fat: 17g
- Carbs: 6g
- Fiber: 2g
- Sugars: 2g

Tips:
- For a lighter option, you can use egg whites or a combination of whole eggs and egg whites.
- Fresh herbs such as parsley or chives can be added for extra flavor without overwhelming sensitivity.

5. Coconut Yogurt Parfait with Strawberries

Preparation Time:
- 5 minutes
- Serves: 2

Ingredients:
- 1 cup coconut yogurt (unsweetened)
- 1/2 cup fresh strawberries, sliced
- 1 tablespoon chia seeds
- 1 tablespoon unsweetened shredded coconut (optional)

Instructions:

1. In two small bowls or glasses, layer coconut yogurt, sliced strawberries, and chia seeds.
2. Top with shredded coconut for an extra texture (optional).
3. Serve immediately or refrigerate for a cool breakfast.

Nutritional Value (per serving):

- Calories: 150
- Protein: 4g
- Fat: 10g
- Carbs: 15g
- Fiber: 4g
- Sugars: 8g

Tips:

- If you're sensitive to coconut, substitute coconut yogurt with a gentle dairy-free option like almond or oat-based yogurt.
- Adjust the sweetness by adding a touch of honey or maple syrup if preferred.

6. Avocado Toast on Gluten-Free Bread

Preparation Time:
- 10 minutes
- Servings: 4

Ingredients:
- 4 slices gluten-free bread
- 2 ripe avocados
- 1 tbsp olive oil
- 1 tsp sea salt
- 1 tsp freshly ground black pepper (optional)
- 1 tbsp fresh lemon juice
- Fresh parsley or cilantro for garnish (optional)

Instructions:
1. Toast the gluten-free bread slices to your desired level of crispness.
2. While the bread is toasting, scoop the avocado flesh into a bowl.

3. Mash the avocados with a fork, adding olive oil, lemon juice, sea salt, and pepper to taste.
4. Spread the mashed avocado mixture evenly over the toasted bread.
5. Garnish with fresh parsley or cilantro, if desired.

Nutritional Value (per serving):
- Calories: ~250
- Carbs: 24g
- Protein: 4g
- Fat: 18g
- Fiber: 8g

Tips:
- Choose gluten-free bread with minimal additives for a healthier option.
- Make sure the avocados are ripe for easier mashing and better flavor.
- Add a drizzle of olive oil to increase the healthy fat content if needed.

7. Rice Pudding with Cinnamon and Honey

Preparation Time:
- 30 minutes
- Servings: 4

Ingredients:
- 1 cup short-grain rice (such as Arborio rice)
- 3 cups unsweetened almond milk (or rice milk)
- 1 tsp cinnamon
- 1 tbsp honey (or to taste)
- 1/2 tsp vanilla extract
- Pinch of sea salt

Instructions:
1. Rinse the rice thoroughly to remove excess starch.
2. In a medium pot, combine the rice, almond milk, and a pinch of salt. Bring to a gentle simmer.

3. Stir occasionally and cook until the rice is soft and the mixture thickens, about 20-25 minutes.
4. Stir in the cinnamon, honey, and vanilla extract, adjusting the sweetness to taste.
5. Serve warm or chilled. Optionally, sprinkle more cinnamon on top before serving.

Nutritional Value (per serving):
- Calories: ~180
- Carbs: 35g
- Protein: 3g
- Fat: 4g
- Fiber: 1g

Tips:
- For extra creaminess, use a bit more almond milk if needed while cooking.
- Adjust the sweetness level by adding more or less honey based on your preference.

8. Banana Nut Smoothie

Preparation Time:
- 5 minutes
- Servings: 4

Ingredients:
- 2 ripe bananas
- 1/2 cup unsweetened almond milk
- 1/4 cup raw walnuts (or almonds)
- 1 tbsp chia seeds (optional)
- 1 tsp honey or maple syrup (optional)
- Ice cubes (optional)

Instructions:
1. Place the bananas, almond milk, walnuts, chia seeds, and honey (if using) into a blender.
2. Blend until smooth, adding ice cubes for a thicker texture if desired.
3. Pour into glasses and serve immediately.

Nutritional Value (per serving):
- Calories: ~200

- Carbs: 30g
- Protein: 4g
- Fat: 9g
- Fiber: 5g

Tips:

- If you prefer a dairy-free version, make sure to choose a plant-based milk without added sugars.
- Walnuts are a great source of omega-3 fatty acids, but you can swap them for other nuts if preferred.

9. Sweet Potato Hash

Preparation Time:
- 25 minutes
- Servings: 4

Ingredients:
- 2 medium sweet potatoes, peeled and diced
- 1 tbsp olive oil
- 1/2 onion, finely chopped
- 1/2 red bell pepper, diced (optional)
- 1 tsp ground cumin
- 1/2 tsp smoked paprika
- 1/4 tsp sea salt
- Fresh cilantro for garnish (optional)

Instructions:
1. Heat olive oil in a large skillet over medium heat.
2. Add the diced sweet potatoes and cook, stirring occasionally, for 10-15 minutes until tender.

3. Add the chopped onion and bell pepper (if using), and cook for an additional 5 minutes.

4. Sprinkle in the cumin, paprika, and sea salt. Stir to combine and cook for another 5 minutes until everything is well-cooked.

5. Garnish with fresh cilantro if desired and serve warm.

Nutritional Value (per serving):
- Calories: ~180
- Carbs: 36g
- Protein: 3g
- Fat: 5g
- Fiber: 6g

Tips:
- You can make this hash with any seasonal root vegetables you have available.
- Make sure the sweet potatoes are tender before serving; you can cover the skillet with a lid to speed up cooking.

10. Apple Cinnamon Quinoa

Preparation Time:
- 20 minutes
- Servings: 4

Ingredients:
- 1 cup quinoa, rinsed
- 2 cups water or unsweetened apple juice
- 1 medium apple, diced
- 1 tsp cinnamon
- 1 tbsp honey or maple syrup (optional)
- 1/4 cup chopped walnuts (optional)

Instructions:
1. In a medium pot, combine quinoa and water (or apple juice). Bring to a boil.
2. Reduce heat to low, cover, and simmer for about 15 minutes until the quinoa is tender and the liquid is absorbed.
3. While the quinoa is cooking, sauté the diced apple in a small skillet with a bit of water over medium heat for about 5 minutes until soft.

4. Stir the sautéed apple, cinnamon, and honey (if using) into the cooked quinoa. Mix well.
5. Optionally, top with chopped walnuts before serving.

Nutritional Value (per serving):
- Calories: ~220
- Carbs: 40g
- Protein: 6g
- Fat: 5g
- Fiber: 5g

Tips:
- To enhance the flavor, use fresh apple juice for cooking the quinoa.
- You can also swap the apple for pears or berries depending on what's in season.

Chapter 2

Nutritious Salads & Light Meals

In this chapter, I'll walk you through how to make a variety of tasty salads and light meals, thoughtfully designed to be easy on your digestive system while providing essential nutrition. The recipes emphasize fresh, wholesome ingredients, ensuring they are both nourishing and gentle. You'll discover how to prepare colorful, flavorful dishes that are simple to make and crafted to promote your overall health. Get ready to enjoy meals that are not only delicious but also beneficial for your well-being!

1. Spinach & Chicken Salad with Olive Oil Vinaigrette

Preparation Time:
- 15 minutes
- Servings: 6

Ingredients:
- 6 cups fresh spinach leaves
- 2 cooked chicken breasts, sliced
- 1 avocado, diced
- 1/4 cup extra virgin olive oil
- 1 tbsp lemon juice
- 1 tsp honey (optional)
- Salt and pepper to taste

Instructions:
1. In a large bowl, toss together the spinach, avocado, and sliced chicken.
2. In a small bowl, whisk together olive oil, lemon juice, honey, salt, and pepper until emulsified.

3. Drizzle the vinaigrette over the salad and toss to coat evenly.

4. Serve immediately, or refrigerate until ready to serve.

Nutritional Value (per serving):
- Calories: 250
- Protein: 24g
- Fat: 18g
- Carbohydrates: 10g
- Fiber: 5g

Tips:
- Choose chicken that is grilled or baked to avoid any added spices or preservatives.
- To keep the salad fresh longer, store the dressing separately and add just before serving.

2. Grilled Salmon Salad with Avocado

Preparation Time:
- 20 minutes
- Servings: 6

Ingredients:
- 6 oz salmon fillets (about 2 per serving)
- 1 avocado, sliced
- 5 cups mixed greens (such as romaine, butter lettuce, and arugula)
- 2 tbsp olive oil
- 1 tbsp fresh lemon juice
- Salt and pepper to taste

Instructions:
1. Preheat the grill to medium-high heat.
2. Brush the salmon fillets with olive oil, season with salt and pepper, and grill for 4-5 minutes per side, until cooked through.

3. While the salmon is grilling, prepare the salad base by combining mixed greens and sliced avocado in a large bowl.
4. Once the salmon is cooked, flake it into bite-sized pieces and add it to the salad.
5. Drizzle the lemon juice over the salad and toss gently.

Nutritional Value (per serving):
- Calories: 320
- Protein: 28g
- Fat: 21g
- Carbohydrates: 8g
- Fiber: 7g

Tips:
- You can substitute grilled chicken or turkey for the salmon if preferred.
- Ensure the avocado is ripe for the best texture and flavor.

3. Carrot & Cucumber Ribbon Salad

Preparation Time:
- 10 minutes
- Servings: 6

Ingredients:
- 4 medium carrots, peeled and shaved into ribbons
- 1 cucumber, peeled and shaved into ribbons
- 1 tbsp olive oil
- 1 tbsp white vinegar
- 1/2 tsp honey (optional)
- Salt to taste

Instructions:
1. Using a vegetable peeler or mandolin, shave the carrots and cucumber into long ribbons.
2. In a small bowl, whisk together olive oil, vinegar, honey, and salt.

3. Toss the ribbons with the dressing until evenly coated.

4. Serve chilled or at room temperature.

Nutritional Value (per serving):
- Calories: 50
- Protein: 1g
- Fat: 3g
- Carbohydrates: 9g
- Fiber: 3g

Tips:
- This salad pairs well with grilled meats for added protein.
- You can add fresh herbs like parsley or dill for extra flavor.

4. Roasted Beetroot Salad with Arugula

Preparation Time:
- 25 minutes
- Servings: 6

Ingredients:
- 4 medium beets, peeled and cubed
- 2 tbsp olive oil
- Salt and pepper to taste
- 5 cups arugula
- 1 tbsp balsamic vinegar
- 1/4 cup feta cheese (optional)

Instructions:
1. Preheat the oven to 400°F (200°C).
2. Toss the beetroot cubes in olive oil, salt, and pepper, and roast for 20-25 minutes, until tender.
3. In a large bowl, toss the arugula with the roasted beets and balsamic vinegar.

4. If desired, sprinkle with feta cheese before serving.

Nutritional Value (per serving):
- Calories: 120
- Protein: 3g
- Fat: 7g
- Carbohydrates: 15g
- Fiber: 4g

Tips:
- Beets can stain, so wear gloves when peeling and handling them.
- Roasting the beets in advance makes the salad quicker to assemble later.

5. Quinoa & Veggie Power Salad

Preparation Time:
- 20 minutes
- Servings: 6

Ingredients:
- 1 cup quinoa, cooked
- 1 cup steamed broccoli florets
- 1/2 cup red bell pepper, diced
- 1/2 cup zucchini, diced
- 1 tbsp olive oil
- 1 tbsp lemon juice
- Salt and pepper to taste

Instructions:
1. Cook the quinoa according to package instructions, then let it cool.
2. In a large bowl, combine quinoa, broccoli, bell pepper, and zucchini.
3. Drizzle olive oil and lemon juice over the salad, and season with salt and pepper.

4. Toss well to combine.

Nutritional Value (per serving):
- Calories: 180
- Protein: 6g
- Fat: 6g
- Carbohydrates: 26g
- Fiber: 5g

Tips:
- For added protein, try adding grilled chicken or tofu.
- Use a variety of colorful vegetables for a nutrient-packed salad.

6. Chopped Cabbage Salad with Lemon Dressing

Preparation Time:
- 15 minutes
- Servings: 3

Ingredients:
- 2 cups of finely chopped green cabbage
- 1 small cucumber, thinly sliced
- 1/4 cup shredded carrots
- 2 tbsp olive oil
- 1 tbsp lemon juice (freshly squeezed)
- 1/2 tsp honey (optional)
- A pinch of salt (optional, based on preference)

Instructions:
1. In a large mixing bowl, combine the cabbage, cucumber, and shredded carrots.
2. In a small bowl, whisk together the olive oil, lemon juice, honey, and a pinch of salt until well combined.

3. Pour the dressing over the salad and toss gently to coat.
4. Serve immediately or refrigerate for up to 2 hours for flavors to meld.

Nutritional Value (per serving):
- Calories: 110
- Carbohydrates: 10g
- Protein: 1g
- Fat: 8g
- Fiber: 3g
- Vitamin A: 70% DV
- Vitamin C: 40% DV

Tips:
- Use a mild cabbage variety like napa cabbage if you prefer a less bitter taste.
- For a bit of crunch, add sunflower seeds or pumpkin seeds if tolerated.

7. Turkey & Cranberry Spinach Salad

Preparation Time:
- 10 minutes
- Servings: 3

Ingredients:
- 3 cups fresh spinach, washed and torn
- 1/2 cup cooked turkey breast, sliced or shredded (preferably without skin or seasoning)
- 2 tbsp fresh cranberries (or dried, unsweetened if preferred)
- 1 tbsp olive oil
- 1 tbsp apple cider vinegar
- 1 tsp honey (optional)

Instructions:
1. In a large bowl, toss together the spinach, turkey, and cranberries.

2. In a separate small bowl, mix the olive oil, apple cider vinegar, and honey until well combined.
3. Drizzle the dressing over the salad and toss gently.
4. Serve immediately.

Nutritional Value (per serving):
- Calories: 150
- Carbohydrates: 10g
- Protein: 20g
- Fat: 7g
- Fiber: 4g
- Vitamin A: 70% DV
- Vitamin K: 50% DV

Tips:
- If fresh cranberries are too tart, try a small amount of apple slices instead.
- Avoid adding nuts or seeds if you're looking to keep the dish very gentle.

8. Roasted Sweet Potato & Kale Salad

Preparation Time:
- 30 minutes (includes roasting time)
- Servings: 3

Ingredients:
- 2 medium sweet potatoes, peeled and cubed
- 4 cups kale, chopped (remove tough stems)
- 2 tbsp olive oil
- 1 tbsp lemon juice
- 1/4 tsp ground cinnamon (optional)
- A pinch of salt

Instructions:
1. Preheat the oven to 400°F (200°C).
2. Toss the sweet potato cubes with 1 tbsp of olive oil, cinnamon, and a pinch of salt. Spread them out on a baking sheet and roast for 20-25 minutes, turning halfway, until tender.

3. Meanwhile, massage the kale with 1 tbsp olive oil and lemon juice for 2-3 minutes to soften the leaves.
4. Once the sweet potatoes are done, let them cool slightly and then toss them with the kale.
5. Serve warm or chilled.

Nutritional Value (per serving):
- Calories: 180
- Carbohydrates: 34g
- Protein: 3g
- Fat: 7g
- Fiber: 6g
- Vitamin A: 180% DV
- Vitamin C: 30% DV

Tips:
- If kale is too tough, you can substitute with a more tender green like spinach.
- Add roasted chicken for extra protein if desired.

9. Simple Avocado & Tomato Salad

Preparation Time:
- 10 minutes
- Servings: 3

Ingredients:
- 2 ripe avocados, diced
- 1 cup cherry tomatoes, halved
- 1 tbsp olive oil
- 1 tbsp lemon juice
- Fresh basil leaves, chopped (optional)
- A pinch of salt

Instructions:
1. In a medium bowl, combine the diced avocado and halved cherry tomatoes.
2. Drizzle the olive oil and lemon juice over the salad.
3. Toss gently to mix, being careful not to mash the avocado.

4. Garnish with fresh basil if desired, and serve immediately.

Nutritional Value (per serving):
- Calories: 240
- Carbohydrates: 12g
- Protein: 3g
- Fat: 22g
- Fiber: 8g
- Vitamin E: 15% DV
- Potassium: 20% DV

Tips:
- To make this dish more filling, add grilled chicken or turkey breast.
- For extra flavor, sprinkle a little ground pepper, if tolerated.

10. Zucchini Noodles with Lemon

Preparation Time:
- 10 minutes
- Servings: 3

Ingredients:
- 3 medium zucchinis, spiralized into noodles
- 2 tbsp olive oil
- 1 tbsp lemon juice
- Zest of 1 lemon
- 1 clove garlic, minced (optional, based on tolerance)
- A pinch of salt

Instructions:
1. Heat olive oil in a skillet over medium heat.
2. Add the garlic (if using) and sauté for 1-2 minutes until fragrant.

3. Add the zucchini noodles and cook for 3-4 minutes, stirring occasionally until tender but still al dente.

4. Remove from heat and stir in the lemon juice, zest, and a pinch of salt.

5. Serve immediately, garnished with fresh herbs if desired.

Nutritional Value (per serving):
- Calories: 120
- Carbohydrates: 10g
- Protein: 2g
- Fat: 9g
- Fiber: 4g
- Vitamin C: 30% DV
- Vitamin A: 25% DV

Tips:
- If you prefer softer noodles, cook them a bit longer.
- Add grilled chicken or shrimp for a protein boost.

Chapter 3

Hearty Soups & Stews

Chapter 3, Hearty Soups & Stews, features a variety of comforting, flavorful recipes tailored for the IC (Interstitial Cystitis) diet. Each dish is crafted to steer clear of common bladder irritants, emphasizing soothing, anti-inflammatory ingredients such as tender vegetables, lean proteins, and mild seasonings. These nourishing soups and stews offer warmth and comfort while being gentle on the bladder, providing a satisfying, symptom-friendly meal. Designed with the IC diet in mind, this chapter ensures you can enjoy hearty, fulfilling dishes without discomfort.

1. Creamy Carrot & Ginger Soup

Preparation Time:
- 30 minutes
- Serves: 2

Ingredients:
- 4 medium carrots, peeled and chopped
- 1 tablespoon fresh ginger, grated
- 1 tablespoon olive oil
- 2 cups low-sodium vegetable broth
- 1/2 cup unsweetened coconut milk
- Salt (optional, to taste)
- Fresh parsley for garnish (optional)

Instructions:
1. Heat the olive oil in a large pot over medium heat. Add the grated ginger and sauté for 1-2 minutes until fragrant.
2. Add the chopped carrots and vegetable broth. Bring to a boil and then lower the heat. Simmer

for 15-20 minutes, or until the carrots are tender.
3. Use an immersion blender to blend the soup until smooth, or transfer to a blender in batches.
4. Stir in the coconut milk and season with salt (if desired). Heat for an additional 5 minutes.
5. Serve warm, garnished with fresh parsley if desired.

Nutritional Value (per serving):
- Calories: 160
- Protein: 2g
- Carbs: 23g
- Fat: 7g
- Fiber: 5g

Tips:
- Adjust the ginger to taste depending on your preference for spiciness.
- You can substitute coconut milk with a lactose-free option if needed.

2. Chicken & Vegetable Broth

Preparation Time:
- 40 minutes
- Serves: 2

Ingredients:
- 2 skinless, boneless chicken breasts
- 4 cups water
- 1 small zucchini, sliced
- 1 small carrot, peeled and sliced
- 1/2 celery stalk, chopped
- 1/2 small onion, chopped
- 1 teaspoon olive oil
- 1 bay leaf
- Salt (optional, to taste)

Instructions:

1. Heat the olive oil in a large pot over medium heat. Add the chopped onion and sauté for 2 minutes.
2. Add the chicken breasts to the pot, followed by the water, carrots, zucchini, celery, bay leaf, and a pinch of salt (optional).
3. Bring to a boil, then reduce heat to low and simmer for 30 minutes, or until the chicken is cooked through and vegetables are tender.
4. Remove the chicken, shred it, and return it to the pot.
5. Discard the bay leaf and adjust seasoning as needed before serving.

Nutritional Value (per serving):

- Calories: 210
- Protein: 28g
- Carbs: 12g
- Fat: 8g
- Fiber: 2g

Tips:
- For a clearer broth, strain before serving.
- Add mild herbs like thyme or parsley for extra flavor.

3. Butternut Squash Soup with Coconut Milk

Preparation Time:
- 45 minutes
- Serves: 2

Ingredients:
- 2 cups cubed butternut squash
- 1 tablespoon olive oil
- 1 small onion, chopped
- 2 cups low-sodium vegetable broth
- 1/2 cup unsweetened coconut milk
- 1/2 teaspoon ground turmeric (optional)
- Salt (optional, to taste)

Instructions:

1. Heat olive oil in a large pot over medium heat. Add the chopped onion and sauté for 5 minutes until softened.
2. Add the cubed butternut squash, vegetable broth, and turmeric (if using). Bring to a boil, then reduce heat and simmer for 25-30 minutes, or until the squash is tender.
3. Blend the soup until smooth using an immersion blender or a regular blender.
4. Stir in the coconut milk and season with salt (if desired). Warm for an additional 5 minutes.
5. Serve warm.

Nutritional Value (per serving):
- Calories: 210
- Protein: 2g
- Carbs: 36g
- Fat: 8g
- Fiber: 7g

Tips:
- If you prefer a thicker soup, reduce the amount of broth or add extra squash.
- Adding a pinch of cinnamon can provide a warming touch without overpowering the flavor.

4. Potato Leek Soup

Preparation Time:
- 45 minutes
- Serves: 2

Ingredients:
- 2 medium potatoes, peeled and diced
- 1 leek, cleaned and chopped
- 1 tablespoon olive oil
- 2 cups low-sodium vegetable broth
- 1/2 cup lactose-free milk (or preferred dairy alternative)
- Salt (optional, to taste)

Instructions:

1. Heat olive oil in a pot over medium heat. Add the chopped leek and sauté for 5 minutes until soft.
2. Add the diced potatoes and vegetable broth. Bring to a boil, then reduce heat and simmer for 20-25 minutes until the potatoes are tender.
3. Use an immersion blender to blend the soup until smooth, or blend in batches.
4. Stir in the lactose-free milk and season with salt (if desired).
5. Serve warm.

Nutritional Value (per serving):
- Calories: 230
- Protein: 4g
- Carbs: 41g
- Fat: 6g
- Fiber: 4g

Tips:
- If you want a chunkier texture, reserve some of the cooked potatoes and stir them back into the soup after blending.
- You can substitute the leek with green onions for a milder flavor.

5. Lentil & Spinach Stew

Preparation Time:
- 50 minutes
- Serves: 2

Ingredients:
- 1/2 cup dried red lentils, rinsed
- 2 cups fresh spinach, chopped
- 1 tablespoon olive oil
- 1 small carrot, peeled and chopped
- 1 small zucchini, chopped
- 2 cups low-sodium vegetable broth
- 1 teaspoon ground cumin (optional)
- Salt (optional, to taste)

Instructions:

1. Heat olive oil in a pot over medium heat. Add the chopped carrot and zucchini, and sauté for 5 minutes.
2. Add the lentils, vegetable broth, and cumin (if using). Bring to a boil, then reduce heat to low and simmer for 25-30 minutes until the lentils are tender.
3. Stir in the chopped spinach and cook for an additional 5 minutes.
4. Season with salt (if desired) and serve warm.

Nutritional Value (per serving):

- Calories: 220
- Protein: 14g
- Carbs: 38g
- Fat: 4g
- Fiber: 10g

Tips:
- If you prefer a smoother texture, blend half of the stew and mix it back in.
- You can add a squeeze of fresh lemon juice for a bright finish.

6. Sweet Potato & Red Lentil Soup

Preparation Time:
- 40 minutes
- Serves: 6

Ingredients:
- 2 medium sweet potatoes, peeled and diced
- 1 cup red lentils, rinsed
- 1 onion, chopped
- 2 cloves garlic, minced
- 4 cups low-sodium vegetable broth
- 1 tsp ground turmeric
- 1 tsp ground cumin
- 1/2 tsp ground ginger

- 1 tbsp olive oil
- Salt to taste (optional)
- Fresh parsley for garnish (optional)

Instructions:

1. In a large pot, heat olive oil over medium heat. Add onion and garlic, and sauté for about 3-4 minutes until softened.

2. Add sweet potatoes, red lentils, turmeric, cumin, and ginger. Stir to combine.

3. Pour in the vegetable broth and bring to a boil. Reduce heat and let it simmer for 25-30 minutes, or until the sweet potatoes and lentils are tender.

4. Use an immersion blender to puree the soup until smooth. If you prefer a chunkier texture, blend partially.

5. Taste and adjust seasoning with salt if needed.

6. Serve warm, garnished with fresh parsley if desired.

Nutritional Value (per serving):
- Calories: 190
- Protein: 7g
- Carbs: 37g
- Fiber: 7g
- Fat: 3g

Tips:
- Opt for fresh, organic vegetables for a more nutritious and soothing soup.
- You can add a splash of almond milk or coconut milk for a creamier texture.
- Avoid using heavy spices if you're sensitive to certain seasonings.

7. Tomato Basil Soup

Preparation Time:
- 30 minutes
- Serves: 6

Ingredients:
- 6 medium tomatoes, chopped
- 1 small onion, chopped
- 2 cloves garlic, minced
- 3 cups low-sodium vegetable broth
- 1/2 cup fresh basil leaves
- 1 tbsp olive oil
- 1 tsp dried oregano (optional)
- Salt to taste (optional)

Instructions:
1. Heat olive oil in a large pot over medium heat. Add onion and garlic, cooking for about 3-4 minutes.
2. Add chopped tomatoes and cook for another 5 minutes, stirring occasionally.

3. Pour in the vegetable broth, and bring to a simmer. Cook for 10-15 minutes.

4. Add basil leaves and oregano (if using), and blend the soup until smooth using an immersion blender or a regular blender.

5. Taste and add salt as needed. Heat for a few more minutes and serve.

Nutritional Value (per serving):
- Calories: 120
- Protein: 3g
- Carbs: 25g
- Fiber: 5g
- Fat: 3g

Tips:
- For a milder flavor, peel the tomatoes before blending.
- If you want a thicker soup, you can add a small amount of rice flour or cornstarch to the soup.

8. Broccoli & Cauliflower Cream Soup

Preparation Time:
- 30 minutes
- Serves: 6

Ingredients:
- 1 head of broccoli, chopped
- 1 head of cauliflower, chopped
- 1 onion, chopped
- 2 cloves garlic, minced
- 4 cups low-sodium vegetable broth
- 1 tbsp olive oil
- 1/4 cup coconut milk (optional for creaminess)
- Salt and pepper to taste

Instructions:
1. Heat olive oil in a large pot over medium heat. Add onion and garlic and sauté for 3-4 minutes.
2. Add broccoli and cauliflower, cooking for another 5 minutes.

3. Pour in the vegetable broth, bring to a boil, and then simmer for about 20 minutes, or until vegetables are tender.
4. Use an immersion blender to blend the soup until smooth, or transfer to a blender in batches.
5. Stir in coconut milk for extra creaminess (optional), and season with salt and pepper to taste.

Nutritional Value (per serving):
- Calories: 150
- Protein: 5g
- Carbs: 25g
- Fiber: 8g
- Fat: 5g

Tips:

- If you have a sensitive stomach, you can cook the vegetables longer to make them even softer before blending.
- For extra flavor, add a pinch of nutmeg or turmeric.

9. Beef & Root Vegetable Stew

Preparation Time:
- 1 hour
- Serves: 6

Ingredients:
- 1 lb lean beef stew meat, cubed
- 2 carrots, peeled and chopped
- 1 parsnip, peeled and chopped
- 2 potatoes, peeled and diced
- 1 onion, chopped
- 2 cloves garlic, minced
- 4 cups low-sodium beef broth
- 1 tsp dried thyme
- 1 tsp dried rosemary
- 1 tbsp olive oil
- Salt to taste

Instructions:
1. Heat olive oil in a large pot over medium heat. Brown the beef stew meat in batches, removing it once browned.

2. In the same pot, add onion and garlic and sauté for 3-4 minutes.

3. Add carrots, parsnip, and potatoes, stirring to combine.

4. Return the beef to the pot and pour in the beef broth. Add thyme and rosemary.

5. Bring to a boil, then reduce to a simmer and cook for 45 minutes, or until the vegetables are tender and the beef is cooked through.

6. Season with salt to taste, and serve hot.

Nutritional Value (per serving):
- Calories: 300
- Protein: 30g
- Carbs: 35g
- Fiber: 8g
- Fat: 10g

Tips:
- Choose grass-fed beef for a more nutrient-dense option.
- For a richer flavor, let the stew sit for an additional 10 minutes after cooking.

10. Chicken Bone Broth with Carrots

Preparation Time:
- 4-6 hours (slow cooker) or 1 hour (stovetop)
- Serves: 6

Ingredients:
- 4 chicken drumsticks (bone-in)
- 4 carrots, peeled and chopped
- 2 celery stalks, chopped
- 1 onion, chopped
- 1 tbsp apple cider vinegar
- 8 cups filtered water
- 1 tsp dried thyme
- Salt to taste

Instructions:
1. Place the chicken drumsticks, carrots, celery, and onion in a large pot or slow cooker.
2. Add the water and apple cider vinegar (this helps extract the nutrients from the bones).

3. If using a stovetop, bring the mixture to a boil, then reduce heat to low and simmer for 1 hour. If using a slow cooker, cook on low for 4-6 hours.
4. Once cooked, remove the chicken from the broth, discard the bones, and shred the chicken. Return the shredded chicken to the broth.
5. Season with thyme and salt to taste. Serve hot.

Nutritional Value (per serving):
- Calories: 150
- Protein: 18g
- Carbs: 8g
- Fiber: 3g
- Fat: 6g

Tips:
- For a clearer broth, skim off any impurities that rise to the surface during cooking.
- You can freeze the broth in portions for later use.

Chapter 4

Main Dishes for Lunch & Dinner

This chapter features a range of tasty, nutritious, and bladder-friendly main dishes designed specifically for the Interstitial Cystitis (IC) diet. Each recipe is created with low-acid, anti-inflammatory ingredients to help alleviate IC symptoms while still delivering delicious and satisfying meals. With options that include protein-rich choices and vegetable-based dishes, you'll find a variety of meals that won't disrupt your comfort. All recipes are free from common irritants such as citrus, tomatoes, and spicy ingredients, making them perfect for anyone following an IC-conscious diet.

1. Grilled Lemon Herb Chicken with Rice

Preparation Time:

- 30 minutes
- Serves: 6

Ingredients:

- 6 boneless, skinless chicken breasts
- 1 cup jasmine rice (or preferred low-acid rice)
- 2 tbsp olive oil
- 1 lemon (zested and juiced)
- 2 garlic cloves, minced
- 1 tbsp fresh parsley, chopped
- Salt (to taste)
- Freshly ground black pepper (optional)

Instructions:

1. Marinate Chicken: In a bowl, combine olive oil, lemon juice, lemon zest, minced garlic, salt, and pepper. Coat the chicken breasts and marinate for 15-20 minutes.

2. Cook Rice: In a medium saucepan, cook rice according to the package instructions.

3. Grill Chicken: Preheat the grill to medium-high heat. Grill the chicken for 5-7 minutes on each side or until fully cooked.

4. Serve: Plate the rice and top with grilled chicken. Garnish with fresh parsley.

Nutritional Value (per serving):
- Calories: ~250 kcal
- Protein: ~30g
- Carbohydrates: ~20g
- Fat: ~7g

Tips:
- Opt for a mild rice variety like jasmine or basmati to avoid irritation.
- For extra flavor, add a dash of fresh thyme or rosemary to the marinade.
- Be cautious with seasonings like garlic, using it in moderation.

2. Baked Salmon with Steamed Veggies

Preparation Time:
- 25 minutes
- Serves: 6

Ingredients:
- 6 salmon fillets (skin-on or skinless)
- 2 tbsp olive oil
- 1 tsp dried dill
- 1 tbsp lemon zest
- 2 cups broccoli florets
- 2 carrots, sliced
- Salt (to taste)
- Freshly ground black pepper (optional)

Instructions:
1. Prepare Salmon: Preheat the oven to 375°F (190°C). Place the salmon fillets on a baking sheet. Drizzle with olive oil, sprinkle with dill, lemon zest, salt, and pepper.

2. Bake Salmon: Bake for 15-18 minutes, until the salmon is cooked through and flakes easily.

3. Steam Veggies: In a steamer or pot with a steam basket, steam the broccoli and carrots for about 5-7 minutes, or until tender.

4. Serve: Plate the baked salmon with the steamed veggies.

Nutritional Value (per serving):
- Calories: ~300 kcal
- Protein: ~30g
- Carbohydrates: ~10g
- Fat: ~18g

Tips:
- Opt for mild herbs like dill or parsley to keep the flavor subtle and soothing.
- Avoid using heavy oils or butter that could irritate.
- Steamed vegetables like carrots and broccoli are easy on digestion and nourishing.

3. Veggie-Stuffed Bell Peppers

Preparation Time:
- 35 minutes
- Serves: 6

Ingredients:
- 6 bell peppers (any color)
- 1 cup cooked quinoa
- 1 cup zucchini, finely diced
- 1 cup spinach, chopped
- 1/2 cup shredded mozzarella cheese (optional)
- 1 tbsp olive oil
- Salt (to taste)
- Freshly ground black pepper (optional)

Instructions:

1. Prepare Peppers: Preheat the oven to 375°F (190°C). Slice the tops off the bell peppers and remove seeds. Place the peppers in a baking dish.

2. Cook Filling: In a pan, heat olive oil over medium heat. Add zucchini and spinach, cooking for 5 minutes until soft.

3. Stuff Peppers: Mix the cooked quinoa with the veggie mixture. Stuff the bell peppers with the quinoa-veggie mixture and top with cheese, if using.

4. Bake: Cover with foil and bake for 20-25 minutes. Remove the foil for the last 5 minutes to allow the cheese to melt.

5. Serve: Remove from the oven and serve warm.

Nutritional Value (per serving):

- Calories: ~220 kcal
- Protein: ~7g
- Carbohydrates: ~30g
- Fat: ~8g

Tips:
- Bell peppers are mild and non-irritating, making them a great base for this dish.
- If you want to lower the fat content, omit the cheese.
- Use mild herbs like basil or oregano for flavor.

4. Zucchini Noodles with Chicken & Olive Oil

Preparation Time:
- 20 minutes
- Serves: 6

Ingredients:
- 3 medium zucchini (spiralized into noodles)
- 4 boneless, skinless chicken breasts, sliced thin
- 2 tbsp olive oil
- 1 tsp dried oregano
- 1 tbsp lemon juice

- 1 tbsp fresh basil, chopped
- Salt (to taste)

Instructions:

1. Cook Chicken: Heat olive oil in a skillet over medium heat. Add the sliced chicken breasts and cook for 5-7 minutes until golden and cooked through. Sprinkle with oregano and salt.

2. Prepare Zucchini Noodles: In the same skillet, add the zucchini noodles and sauté for 2-3 minutes until tender but still crisp.

3. Combine: Add the cooked chicken back to the skillet and toss together with the zucchini noodles. Drizzle with lemon juice and top with fresh basil.

4. Serve: Plate the zucchini noodles with chicken and serve immediately.

Nutritional Value (per serving):

- Calories: ~230 kcal
- Protein: ~30g
- Carbohydrates: ~10g
- Fat: ~10g

Tips:
- Zucchini noodles are a great alternative to pasta and are very gentle on digestion.
- For a richer flavor, you can add a small amount of grated Parmesan (optional).

5. Turkey Meatballs with Quinoa

Preparation Time:
- 40 minutes
- Serves: 6

Ingredients:
- 1 lb ground turkey
- 1/2 cup cooked quinoa
- 1/4 cup fresh parsley, chopped
- 1 egg
- 1 tbsp olive oil
- Salt (to taste)
- Freshly ground black pepper (optional)

Instructions:

1. Prepare Meatballs: Preheat oven to 375°F (190°C). In a large bowl, mix the ground turkey, cooked quinoa, parsley, egg, salt, and pepper.

2. Form Meatballs: Roll the mixture into small meatballs, about 1-inch in diameter, and place them on a baking sheet.

3. Bake: Drizzle with olive oil and bake for 20-25 minutes until fully cooked and golden brown.

4. Serve: Serve warm with a side of steamed vegetables or over a bed of quinoa.

Nutritional Value (per serving):

- Calories: ~220 kcal
- Protein: ~25g
- Carbohydrates: ~15g
- Fat: ~10g

Tips:
- Ground turkey is a lean protein that is easy to digest.
- Quinoa is rich in fiber and adds a wholesome base for the meatballs.
- You can also add a small amount of grated carrot to the meatball mixture for added nutrition.

6. Grilled Cod with Sweet Potato Mash

Preparation Time:
- 25 minutes
- Serves: 2

Ingredients:
- 2 cod fillets
- 1 medium sweet potato, peeled and cubed
- 1 tbsp olive oil
- 1 tsp fresh thyme (optional)
- Salt (to taste)

- Fresh ground pepper (optional, for a mild taste)
- 1 tbsp unsweetened almond milk (or any non-dairy milk)
- 1 tbsp butter (or substitute with olive oil)

Instructions:

1. Grill the Cod: Preheat the grill to medium heat. Season the cod fillets lightly with olive oil and fresh thyme. Grill for 4-5 minutes on each side until cooked through.

2. Make the Sweet Potato Mash: While the cod is grilling, place the cubed sweet potato in a pot of boiling water. Cook until tender (about 10 minutes). Drain and mash with almond milk and butter until smooth. Add salt to taste.

3. Serve: Plate the grilled cod with a generous serving of mashed sweet potatoes on the side.

Nutritional Value (per serving):
- Calories: ~220 kcal
- Protein: ~22g
- Carbohydrates: ~30g
- Fat: ~5g
- Fiber: ~4g

Tips:
- For extra flavor, try adding a squeeze of lemon to the cod before serving.
- Ensure that the cod is fresh and not heavily seasoned with any acidic ingredients (like lemon or vinegar) to avoid irritation.

7. Eggplant Parmesan

Preparation Time:
- 35 minutes
- Serves: 2

Ingredients:
- 1 medium eggplant, sliced into ½-inch thick rounds
- ½ cup gluten-free breadcrumbs (or panko)
- 1 egg (beaten)
- ½ cup mozzarella cheese, shredded
- 1 tbsp olive oil
- Salt (to taste)
- Fresh basil for garnish (optional)

Instructions:
1. Prep Eggplant: Preheat the oven to 375°F (190°C). Arrange the eggplant slices on a baking sheet, brush each side with olive oil, and sprinkle with salt. Bake for 15-20 minutes until soft and lightly golden.

2. Coat the Eggplant: In a shallow dish, dip the eggplant rounds into the beaten egg, then coat with gluten-free breadcrumbs.

3. Assemble: Once all eggplant slices are coated, layer them in a baking dish. Top each slice with shredded mozzarella cheese.

4. Bake: Place the baking dish in the oven and bake for an additional 10 minutes or until the cheese is melted and bubbly.

5. Serve: Garnish with fresh basil and serve warm.

Nutritional Value (per serving):
- Calories: ~250 kcal
- Protein: ~12g
- Carbohydrates: ~24g
- Fat: ~15g
- Fiber: ~6g

Tips:
- For a lighter version, try skipping the cheese or using a dairy-free alternative.
- You can also sauté the eggplant slices in a non-stick pan with a little olive oil instead of baking them.

8 Roasted Chicken with Green Beans

Preparation Time:
- 40 minutes
- Serves: 2

Ingredients:
- 2 chicken breasts (boneless, skinless)
- 1 tbsp olive oil
- 1 tsp rosemary (optional)
- Salt and mild pepper (to taste)
- 2 cups green beans (trimmed)
- 1 tbsp butter (optional for the green beans)

Instructions:

1. Roast the Chicken: Preheat the oven to 375°F (190°C). Rub the chicken breasts with olive oil, rosemary, and salt. Roast for 25-30 minutes or until the internal temperature reaches 165°F (74°C).

2. Cook the Green Beans: While the chicken is roasting, steam the green beans until tender, about 5-7 minutes. Toss with a little butter and salt (optional).

3. Serve: Plate the roasted chicken alongside the steamed green beans for a balanced meal.

Nutritional Value (per serving):

- Calories: ~280 kcal
- Protein: ~40g
- Carbohydrates: ~10g
- Fat: ~12g
- Fiber: ~4g

Tips:
- Use a meat thermometer to ensure the chicken is properly cooked.
- Green beans can be sautéed in olive oil for added flavor.

9. Baked Tilapia with Sautéed Spinach

Preparation Time:
- 20 minutes
- Serves: 2

Ingredients:
- 2 tilapia fillets
- 1 tbsp olive oil
- 1 clove garlic (optional, finely minced)
- 4 cups fresh spinach
- Salt to taste
- Fresh lemon wedges (optional)

Instructions:

1. Bake the Tilapia: Preheat the oven to 375°F (190°C). Season the tilapia fillets with olive oil and a pinch of salt. Bake for 12-15 minutes or until the fish flakes easily.

2. Sauté the Spinach: While the tilapia is baking, heat a pan with a little olive oil. Add the minced garlic (if using) and sauté for 1 minute. Add the spinach and cook until wilted, about 2-3 minutes. Season with salt.

3. Serve: Plate the tilapia with a side of sautéed spinach and garnish with a fresh lemon wedge if desired.

Nutritional Value (per serving):

- Calories: ~180 kcal
- Protein: ~22g
- Carbohydrates: ~6g
- Fat: ~8g
- Fiber: ~3g

Tips:
- To avoid potential irritants, use garlic sparingly or omit it altogether if necessary.
- For added flavor, try a dash of mild olive oil or a sprinkle of fresh herbs.

10. Quinoa & Vegetable Stir-Fry

Preparation Time:
- 30 minute
- Serves: 2

Ingredients:
- 1 cup quinoa (cooked according to package instructions)
- 1 cup bell peppers (diced)
- 1 medium zucchini (sliced)
- ½ cup carrots (sliced thin)
- 2 tbsp olive oil
- 1 tbsp tamari or low-sodium soy sauce (optional)
- Salt and pepper to taste

Instructions:

1. Cook the Quinoa: Cook quinoa according to the package instructions and set aside.

2. Sauté the Vegetables: Heat olive oil in a pan over medium heat. Add the bell peppers, zucchini, and carrots. Cook for 5-7 minutes until tender but still slightly crisp.

3. Combine: Add the cooked quinoa to the pan with the vegetables and stir-fry for another 2-3 minutes. Season with tamari (optional), salt, and pepper.

4. Serve: Serve the stir-fry warm, topped with fresh herbs if desired.

Nutritional Value (per serving):
- Calories: ~250 kcal
- Protein: ~8g
- Carbohydrates: ~40g
- Fat: ~9g
- Fiber: ~5g

Tips:

- Feel free to swap vegetables based on your preferences or what you have on hand.
- For a more filling meal, add a mild protein source like grilled chicken or tofu.

Chapter 5

Sides & Vegetables

Chapter 5: Sides & Vegetables features a selection of vegetable-centric recipes that are soothing for the bladder and suitable for individuals with Interstitial Cystitis (IC). It highlights ingredients that are low in acid and free from typical IC triggers, offering simple, tasty side dishes and vegetable options that promote a healthy, calming diet.

1. Roasted Garlic & Herb Sweet Potatoes

Preparation Time:
- 40 minutes

Ingredients:
- 4 medium sweet potatoes, peeled and cubed
- 2 tbsp olive oil
- 1 tsp dried rosemary
- 1 tsp dried thyme
- 1 tsp garlic powder (or fresh garlic)
- Salt (to taste)
- Fresh parsley (optional, for garnish)

Instructions:
1. Preheat the oven to 400°F (200°C).
2. Toss the cubed sweet potatoes in olive oil, rosemary, thyme, garlic powder, and salt.
3. Spread them on a baking sheet in a single layer.

4. Roast for 30-35 minutes, or until tender and lightly browned, flipping halfway through.
5. Garnish with fresh parsley, if desired.

Nutritional Value (per serving):
- Calories: 150
- Carbohydrates: 35g
- Protein: 2g
- Fat: 3g
- Fiber: 5g

Tips:
- Use fresh herbs if available for more vibrant flavor.
- Keep the garlic portion low to avoid overwhelming sensitivities.

2. Steamed Asparagus with Lemon Zest

Preparation Time:
- 10 minutes

Ingredients:
- 1 bunch asparagus, trimmed
- 1 tbsp olive oil
- 1 tsp lemon zest
- Salt and pepper (to taste)

Instructions:
1. Steam the asparagus in a steamer basket over boiling water for about 5-7 minutes, or until tender but still vibrant green.
2. Remove and drizzle with olive oil.
3. Sprinkle with lemon zest, salt, and pepper to taste.
4. Serve immediately.

Nutritional Value (per serving):
- Calories: 40
- Carbohydrates: 8g
- Protein: 3g
- Fat: 2g
- Fiber: 3g

Tips:
- Avoid overcooking the asparagus to maintain nutrients and texture.
- Lemon zest adds a mild citrus flavor without being overpowering.

3. Sautéed Spinach with Olive Oil & Garlic

Preparation Time:
- 10 minutes

Ingredients:
- 4 cups fresh spinach
- 1 tbsp olive oil
- 1 clove garlic, minced
- Salt to taste

Instructions:
1. Heat olive oil in a large skillet over medium heat.
2. Add the garlic and sauté for about 30 seconds, being careful not to brown.
3. Add the spinach and cook for 2-3 minutes until wilted, stirring occasionally.
4. Season with salt and serve.

Nutritional Value (per serving):
- Calories: 70
- Carbohydrates: 6g
- Protein: 3g
- Fat: 5g
- Fiber: 4g

Tips:
- Spinach cooks down significantly, so feel free to adjust the quantity.
- Fresh garlic should be used sparingly to avoid irritation.

4. Baked Zucchini Fries

Preparation Time:
- 30 minutes

Ingredients:
- 2 medium zucchinis, cut into fry shapes
- 1/2 cup gluten-free breadcrumbs
- 1/4 cup grated parmesan (optional)
- 1 egg (beaten)
- 1 tbsp olive oil
- Salt and pepper to taste

Instructions:
1. Preheat the oven to 425°F (220°C).
2. Dip each zucchini piece into the egg, then coat with breadcrumbs and parmesan (if using).
3. Place them in a single layer on a baking sheet lined with parchment paper.
4. Drizzle with olive oil and bake for 20-25 minutes, flipping halfway through, until crispy and golden.
5. Serve immediately.

Nutritional Value (per serving):
- Calories: 120
- Carbohydrates: 16g
- Protein: 5g
- Fat: 6g
- Fiber: 4g

Tips:
- For extra crunch, you can double-coat the zucchini fries.
- Experiment with different seasonings like oregano or parsley to adjust flavor.

5. Cauliflower Rice Pilaf

Preparation Time:
- 20 minutes

Ingredients:
- 1 head of cauliflower, grated or processed into rice-sized pieces
- 1 tbsp olive oil
- 1/4 cup diced onions (optional, based on tolerance)
- 1/2 cup diced carrots
- 1/4 cup fresh parsley, chopped
- Salt to taste

Instructions:
1. Heat olive oil in a large pan over medium heat.
2. Add the onions and carrots, cooking for about 5 minutes until soft.
3. Add the cauliflower rice and cook for an additional 5-7 minutes, stirring occasionally.

4. Season with salt and garnish with parsley before serving.

Nutritional Value (per serving):
- Calories: 70
- Carbohydrates: 14g
- Protein: 3g
- Fat: 4g
- Fiber: 4g

Tips:
- Cauliflower rice can be prepared ahead of time and stored in the fridge for 2-3 days.
- If avoiding onions, replace them with a small amount of garlic for flavor.

6. Mashed Butternut Squash

Preparation Time:
- 25 minutes

Ingredients:
- 1 medium butternut squash, peeled and cubed
- 1 tbsp olive oil or butter
- 1/4 cup low-sodium vegetable broth (or as needed)
- Salt to taste
- A pinch of nutmeg (optional)

Instructions:
1. Steam or boil the butternut squash until tender, about 15 minutes.
2. Drain and place in a bowl.
3. Mash with a fork or potato masher, adding olive oil or butter and vegetable broth for desired consistency.
4. Season with salt and a pinch of nutmeg if desired, then serve.

Nutritional Value (per serving):

- Calories: 120
- Carbohydrates: 30g
- Protein: 2g
- Fat: 4g
- Fiber: 6g

Tips:

- You can add a bit of cinnamon for warmth if tolerated.
- Adjust the consistency by adding more broth if you prefer a smoother texture.

7. Roasted Brussels Sprouts with Apple Cider Vinegar

Preparation Time:
- 25 minutes
- Serves: 4

Ingredients:
- 1 lb Brussels sprouts, trimmed and halved
- 2 tbsp olive oil
- 1 tbsp apple cider vinegar
- Salt (optional)
- Freshly ground black pepper (optional)

Instructions:
1. Preheat the oven to 400°F (200°C).
2. Toss the halved Brussels sprouts in olive oil until evenly coated.
3. Arrange the Brussels sprouts on a baking sheet in a single layer.
4. Roast for 20-25 minutes or until crispy and golden brown, stirring halfway through.

5. Drizzle apple cider vinegar over the Brussels sprouts and toss to combine.
6. Season with salt and pepper if desired.
7. Serve warm.

Nutritional Value (per serving):
- Calories: 120
- Protein: 4g
- Fat: 10g
- Carbohydrates: 10g
- Fiber: 4g
- Sugars: 3g

Tips:
- For extra flavor, add a sprinkle of fresh herbs like rosemary or thyme before roasting.
- You can substitute apple cider vinegar with a milder vinegar if preferred.

8. Sautéed Green Beans with Almonds

Preparation Time:
- 15 minutes
- Serves: 4

Ingredients:
- 1 lb fresh green beans, trimmed
- 2 tbsp olive oil
- 1/4 cup sliced almonds, toasted
- Salt (optional)
- Freshly ground black pepper (optional)

Instructions:
1. Heat the olive oil in a large skillet over medium heat.
2. Add the green beans and sauté for 6-8 minutes, stirring occasionally, until tender but still crisp.
3. Stir in the toasted almonds and cook for another 1-2 minutes.
4. Season with salt and pepper to taste.

5. Serve warm.

Nutritional Value (per serving):
- Calories: 130
- Protein: 3g
- Fat: 11g
- Carbohydrates: 7g
- Fiber: 3g
- Sugars: 3g

Tips:
- To toast almonds, place them in a dry skillet over medium heat for 2-3 minutes, shaking the pan frequently to prevent burning.
- For a crunchier texture, sauté the green beans a little longer, but be careful not to overcook them.

9. Carrot & Cucumber Sticks with Hummus

Preparation Time:
- 10 minutes
- Serves: 4

Ingredients:
- 3 medium carrots, peeled and cut into sticks
- 1 cucumber, sliced into sticks
- 1 cup homemade or store-bought plain hummus (without garlic or citrus)

Instructions:
1. Arrange the carrot and cucumber sticks on a platter.
2. Serve with a bowl of hummus for dipping.
3. Enjoy immediately.

Nutritional Value (per serving):
- Calories: 100
- Protein: 3g
- Fat: 6g
- Carbohydrates: 12g
- Fiber: 4g
- Sugars: 6g

Tips:

- Use a mild-flavored hummus that doesn't include garlic or lemon for a more soothing experience.
- You can substitute cucumber with zucchini or bell pepper sticks for variety.

10. Grilled Veggie Skewers

Preparation Time:
- 30 minutes
- Serves: 4

Ingredients:
- 1 red bell pepper, cut into chunks
- 1 yellow bell pepper, cut into chunks
- 1 zucchini, sliced
- 1 small red onion, cut into chunks
- 8-10 cherry tomatoes
- 2 tbsp olive oil
- Salt (optional)
- Freshly ground black pepper (optional)
- Fresh herbs like basil or parsley for garnish (optional)

Instructions:
1. Preheat the grill to medium heat.
2. Thread the veggies onto skewers, alternating between peppers, zucchini, onion, and tomatoes.

3. Brush the veggies with olive oil and season with salt and pepper.
4. Grill the skewers for about 8-10 minutes, turning occasionally, until the vegetables are tender and lightly charred.
5. Garnish with fresh herbs if desired and serve.

Nutritional Value (per serving):
- Calories: 140
- Protein: 3g
- Fat: 10g
- Carbohydrates: 14g
- Fiber: 5g
- Sugars: 7g

Tips:
- You can use other vegetables like mushrooms, eggplant, or squash for variety.
- If you're using wooden skewers, soak them in water for 30 minutes before grilling to prevent burning.

Chapter 6

Healthy Snacks & Treats

Chapter 6 is dedicated to offering healthy snack and treat options for managing interstitial cystitis (IC). It provides a variety of recipes crafted with bladder-friendly ingredients, emphasizing those that are low in acidity, free from caffeine, and free from harmful additives. The chapter also incorporates anti-inflammatory ingredients such as turmeric and ginger, which are known to help reduce inflammation. A strong focus is placed on portion control and smart ingredient substitutions. Recipes include delightful options like fruit popsicles, baked zucchini chips, almond protein bars, and many others, all designed to support a balanced, bladder-friendly diet.

1. Turmeric and Ginger Tea

Preparation Time:
- 5 minutes
- Serves: 1

Ingredients:
- 1/2 teaspoon ground turmeric
- 1/2 teaspoon ground ginger
- 1 cup hot water
- Honey (optional)

Instructions:
1. Boil water and pour it into a cup.
2. Stir in the ground turmeric and ginger until well mixed.
3. Add honey if desired for sweetness.
4. Let steep for 2-3 minutes before sipping gently.

Nutritional Value (approx.):
- Calories: 10
- Carbohydrates: 2g
- Protein: 0g
- Fat: 0g
- Fiber: 1g

Tips:
- Avoid adding lemon or acidic ingredients, as they can be irritating.
- Drink this tea once a day to enjoy its anti-inflammatory benefits.

2. Apple Slices with Peanut Butter

Preparation Time:
- 5 minutes
- Serves: 1

Ingredients:
- 1 small apple (peeled, if preferred)
- 1-2 tablespoons peanut butter (unsweetened, natural)

Instructions:
1. Slice the apple into wedges.
2. Spread a thin layer of peanut butter on each slice.
3. Serve immediately or enjoy as a snack.

Nutritional Value (approx. per serving):
- Calories: 150-200 (depending on peanut butter quantity)
- Carbohydrates: 22g
- Protein: 4g
- Fat: 9g
- Fiber: 4g

Tips:
- Choose a peanut butter without added sugar or artificial sweeteners.
- If apples cause irritation, use a pear as an alternative, which is generally milder.

3. Rice Cakes with Avocado Spread

Preparation Time:
- 5 minutes
- Serves: 1

Ingredients:
- 2 plain rice cakes
- 1/2 ripe avocado
- Salt (optional, in moderation)

Instructions:
1. Mash the avocado with a fork until smooth.
2. Spread the mashed avocado evenly over each rice cake.
3. Optionally, sprinkle a pinch of salt on top.
4. Serve immediately.

Nutritional Value (approx. per serving):

- Calories: 150
- Carbohydrates: 20g
- Protein: 2g
- Fat: 9g
- Fiber: 3g

Tips:

- Use plain, unsweetened rice cakes to avoid unnecessary additives.
- If avocado isn't well tolerated, try a mild, seedless cucumber mash as a topping.

4. Cucumber & Cream Cheese Bites

Preparation Time:
- 5 minutes
- Serves: 1

Ingredients:
- 1/2 cucumber
- 2 tablespoons plain cream cheese (lactose-free, if needed)
- Fresh dill or parsley (optional)

Instructions:
1. Slice the cucumber into 1/4-inch thick rounds.
2. Spread a small amount of cream cheese on each cucumber slice.
3. Optionally, top with fresh dill or parsley for added flavor.
4. Serve immediately.

Nutritional Value (approx. per serving):
- Calories: 120
- Carbohydrates: 7g
- Protein: 3g
- Fat: 10g
- Fiber: 2g

Tips:
- Opt for a non-acidic, mild cream cheese to avoid potential irritation.
- For variation, try using a dollop of lactose-free Greek yogurt instead of cream cheese.

5. Carrot Sticks with Tzatziki

Preparation Time:
- 5 minutes
- Serves: 1

Ingredients:
- 1 medium carrot
- 2 tablespoons tzatziki (make sure it's mild and free of garlic or vinegar)

Instructions:
1. Peel and cut the carrot into sticks.
2. Serve with a side of tzatziki for dipping.
3. Enjoy immediately.

Nutritional Value (approx. per serving):
- Calories: 50
- Carbohydrates: 12g
- Protein: 1g
- Fat: 2g
- Fiber: 3g

Tips:
- Choose a homemade or mild store-bought tzatziki, avoiding garlic, vinegar, or lemon for gentler digestion.
- If carrots cause irritation, opt for cucumber or zucchini sticks instead.

6. Baked Zucchini Chips

Preparation Time:
- 15 minutes
- Cooking Time: 25 minutes
- Serves: 2

Ingredients:
- 2 medium zucchinis
- 2 tbsp olive oil
- 1 tsp garlic powder
- 1 tsp dried oregano
- 1/2 tsp salt (or to taste)
- 1/2 tsp black pepper

Instructions:

1. Preheat the oven to 400°F (200°C).
2. Slice zucchinis into thin rounds.
3. In a bowl, toss the zucchini slices with olive oil, garlic powder, oregano, salt, and pepper until well coated.
4. Spread the zucchini slices in a single layer on a baking sheet lined with parchment paper.
5. Bake for 20-25 minutes, flipping halfway through, until crispy.
6. Allow chips to cool for a few minutes before serving.

Nutritional Value (per serving):

- Calories: 150 kcal
- Protein: 2g
- Fat: 14g
- Carbohydrates: 7g
- Fiber: 2g

Tips:
- To prevent sogginess, ensure the zucchini slices are as thin as possible.
- You can also sprinkle a little parmesan cheese after baking for extra flavor.

7. Homemade Popcorn with Olive Oil

Preparation Time:
- 5 minutes
- Cooking Time: 5 minutes
- Serves: 2

Ingredients:
- 1/2 cup popcorn kernels
- 2 tbsp olive oil
- Salt to taste

Instructions:

1. Heat olive oil in a large pot over medium heat.
2. Add popcorn kernels to the pot and cover.
3. Shake the pot occasionally to prevent burning until the popping slows down (around 3-5 minutes).
4. Remove from heat and season with salt before serving.

Nutritional Value (per serving):

- Calories: 120 kcal
- Protein: 3g
- Fat: 8g
- Carbohydrates: 15g
- Fiber: 3g

Tips:

- Experiment with other mild seasonings like dried basil or oregano for variation.
- Air-popped popcorn can also be used for a lower-fat option.

8. Frozen Yogurt Bark with Berries

Preparation Time:
- 10 minutes
- Freezing Time: 2 hours
- Serves: 2

Ingredients:
- 1 cup plain Greek yogurt (unsweetened)
- 1/2 cup fresh blueberries
- 1/2 cup fresh strawberries, sliced
- 1 tbsp honey (optional)

Instructions:
1. Line a baking sheet with parchment paper.
2. Spread Greek yogurt evenly on the sheet, forming a thin layer.
3. Sprinkle the berries evenly over the yogurt.
4. Drizzle honey on top if desired.
5. Freeze for at least 2 hours until solid.
6. Break the bark into pieces and serve.

Nutritional Value (per serving):
- Calories: 120 kcal
- Protein: 7g
- Fat: 3g
- Carbohydrates: 18g
- Fiber: 2g

Tips:
- Use any berries that are gentle on the stomach, such as blueberries and strawberries, and avoid citrus fruits.
- Store any leftovers in an airtight container in the freezer.

9. Coconut Macaroons with Fruit Popsicles

Preparation Time:
- 10 minutes
- Baking Time: 15 minutes
- Serves: 2

Ingredients:
- 1 1/2 cups unsweetened shredded coconut
- 2 large egg whites
- 1/4 cup honey or maple syrup
- 1/2 tsp vanilla extract
- A few fresh berries (optional for topping)

Instructions:
1. Preheat oven to 350°F (175°C).
2. In a bowl, whisk egg whites until soft peaks form.
3. Fold in shredded coconut, honey, and vanilla extract.

4. Scoop spoonfuls of the mixture onto a parchment-lined baking sheet.
5. Bake for 12-15 minutes until golden brown.
6. Let cool before serving. Optional: top with fresh berries.

Nutritional Value (per serving):
- Calories: 180 kcal
- Protein: 3g
- Fat: 12g
- Carbohydrates: 18g
- Fiber: 3g

Tips:
- For added sweetness, you can mix in a little pure maple syrup instead of honey.
- These can be stored in an airtight container for up to a week.

10. Almond Protein Bars

Preparation Time:
- 10 minutes
- Chill Time: 2 hours
- Serves: 2

Ingredients:
- 1 cup almond butter (smooth and unsweetened)
- 1/2 cup rolled oats
- 1/4 cup protein powder (unsweetened)
- 1/4 cup honey or maple syrup
- 1/4 tsp cinnamon
- 1/4 tsp vanilla extract

Instructions:
1. In a bowl, combine almond butter, oats, protein powder, cinnamon, vanilla extract, and honey.
2. Mix until well combined and a dough forms.
3. Press the dough into a lined baking dish and flatten it evenly.

4. Refrigerate for at least 2 hours, then cut into bars.

Nutritional Value (per serving):
- Calories: 220 kcal
- Protein: 8g
- Fat: 16g
- Carbohydrates: 14g
- Fiber: 3g

Tips:
- Store the bars in the fridge to keep them fresh longer.
- Add chopped nuts for an extra crunch, but avoid any irritating seeds.

Chapter 7

Smoothies & Refreshing Beverages

In this chapter, you'll find a variety of soothing, bladder-friendly smoothies and drinks created with the Interstitial Cystitis (IC) diet in mind. Every recipe is thoughtfully designed with gentle, non-irritating ingredients that hydrate, nourish, and refresh, helping you enjoy delicious beverages while avoiding common IC triggers.

1. Green Smoothie with Spinach & Banana

Preparation Time:
- 5 minutes
- Servings: 2

Ingredients:
- 1 cup fresh spinach (organic preferred)
- 1 ripe banana
- 1/2 cup unsweetened almond milk (or any non-dairy milk without added sugars)
- 1/2 cup water
- 1 tbsp ground flax seeds (optional)
- 1-2 ice cubes (optional)

Instructions:
1. Add spinach, banana, almond milk, water, and ground flax seeds (optional) into a blender.
2. Blend until smooth and creamy.
3. Add ice cubes for a chilled effect and blend again until fully incorporated.
4. Pour into glasses and serve immediately.

Nutritional Value (per serving):
- Calories: ~120-140 kcal
- Protein: ~2g
- Carbohydrates: ~30g
- Fat: ~2g
- Fiber: ~3g
- Vitamin A: 56% DV
- Potassium: 400mg
- Calcium: 100mg

Tips:

- Opt for organic spinach to avoid pesticides, which may irritate the bladder.
- Ensure your almond milk is unsweetened, as added sugars can trigger symptoms in some IC patients.
- You may also add 1/2 a pear for natural sweetness.

2. Berry Almond Milk Smoothie

Preparation Time:
- 5 minutes
- Servings: 2

Ingredients:
- 1/2 cup fresh or frozen blueberries (low-acid fruit)
- 1/2 cup fresh or frozen strawberries (if tolerated)
- 1 cup unsweetened almond milk
- 1 tbsp chia seeds (optional for fiber)
- 1/2 tsp honey (optional)
- Ice cubes (optional)

Instructions:
1. Combine the berries, almond milk, chia seeds, and honey (optional) into a blender.
2. Blend until smooth.
3. Add ice cubes to chill the drink and blend again.

4. Pour into glasses and serve immediately.

Nutritional Value (per serving):
- Calories: ~110 kcal
- Protein: ~2g
- Carbohydrates: ~20g
- Fat: ~5g
- Fiber: ~3g
- Vitamin C: 30% DV
- Potassium: 200mg

Tips:
- If strawberries are irritating, replace them with other low-acid fruits such as blueberries or raspberries.
- Always use unsweetened almond milk to avoid added sugars that may aggravate IC symptoms.

3. Tropical Mango Coconut Smoothie

Preparation Time:
- 5 minutes
- Servings: 2

Ingredients:
- 1 cup fresh or frozen mango chunks
- 1/2 cup coconut milk (unsweetened)
- 1/2 cup water
- 1 tbsp ground flaxseed (optional)
- 1 tsp grated ginger (optional)

Instructions:
1. Place the mango, coconut milk, water, flaxseed, and ginger into a blender.
2. Blend until smooth and creamy.
3. Add ice cubes if a colder smoothie is preferred.
4. Pour into glasses and serve immediately.

Nutritional Value (per serving):
- Calories: ~150 kcal
- Protein: ~1g
- Carbohydrates: ~35g
- Fat: ~7g
- Fiber: ~4g
- Vitamin C: 50% DV
- Potassium: 300mg

Tips:
- Avoid canned coconut milk that contains additives or preservatives. Choose a fresh, unsweetened variety.
- Mangoes are a great low-acid fruit but ensure it is ripe to avoid irritation.
- Ground flaxseed can boost omega-3s and fiber, which are gentle on the bladder.

4. Cucumber & Mint Infused Water

Preparation Time:
- 5 minutes (plus 1-2 hours for infusion)
- Servings: 2

Ingredients:
- 1/2 cucumber, thinly sliced
- 1-2 sprigs fresh mint
- 4 cups filtered water
- Ice cubes (optional)

Instructions:
1. Add cucumber slices and mint sprigs to a large pitcher or bottle.
2. Fill with filtered water.
3. Let the water infuse in the fridge for at least 1-2 hours to allow the flavors to develop.
4. Serve chilled over ice if preferred.

Nutritional Value (per serving):
- Calories: ~5 kcal
- Protein: ~0g
- Carbohydrates: ~1g
- Fat: ~0g
- Fiber: ~0g
- Hydration: Excellent

Tips:
- This is a hydrating and soothing drink ideal for IC, as cucumbers are alkaline and mild on the bladder.
- Avoid adding citrus fruits like lemon or lime, which may irritate the bladder.
- Drinking infused water can be a good way to stay hydrated throughout the day.

5. Sweet Carrot & Apple Juice

Preparation Time:
- 5 minutes
- Servings: 2

Ingredients:
- 2 medium carrots, peeled
- 1 small apple (preferably sweet, like Fuji or Gala)
- 1/2 cup water
- 1 tsp ground ginger (optional)

Instructions:
1. Peel the carrots and chop them into smaller pieces.
2. Core and slice the apple.
3. Add carrots, apple, water, and ginger (optional) to a blender.
4. Blend until smooth and pour into a glass.
5. Optionally strain the juice to remove pulp if you prefer a smoother consistency.

Nutritional Value (per serving):
- Calories: ~90 kcal
- Protein: ~1g
- Carbohydrates: ~22g
- Fat: ~0g
- Fiber: ~3g
- Vitamin A: 120% DV
- Potassium: 400mg

Tips:
- Carrots and apples are naturally sweet and IC-friendly, but avoid acidic apples like Granny Smith, which may irritate some individuals.
- Ginger can be a soothing addition if tolerated, but skip it if it causes discomfort.

6. Pear & Ginger Smoothie

Preparation Time:
- 10 minutes
- Serves: 4

Ingredients:
- 2 ripe pears, peeled and cored
- 1-inch piece of fresh ginger, peeled
- 1/2 cup unsweetened almond milk
- 1/2 cup ice cubes
- 1 tablespoon honey (optional)

Instructions:
1. Blend the pears, ginger, and almond milk until smooth.
2. Add ice cubes and honey (if using), then blend again until chilled.
3. Pour into glasses and serve immediately.

Nutritional Value (per serving):
- Calories: 90
- Carbohydrates: 23g
- Protein: 1g
- Fat: 0.5g
- Fiber: 4g
- Sugar: 17g

Tips:
- Ginger can be strong, so adjust the amount based on your preference.
- If you're avoiding sweetness, omit the honey or substitute with a small amount of stevia.

7. Lemon & Honey Detox Drink

Preparation Time:
- 5 minutes
- Serves: 4

Ingredients:
- 1 lemon, juiced
- 4 cups of warm water
- 2 tablespoons honey
- A pinch of fresh mint leaves (optional)

Instructions:
1. In a large pitcher, combine the lemon juice, honey, and warm water.
2. Stir well until the honey is fully dissolved.
3. Garnish with mint leaves if desired.
4. Pour into glasses and serve warm or chilled.

Nutritional Value (per serving):
- Calories: 45
- Carbohydrates: 12g
- Protein: 0g
- Fat: 0g
- Fiber: 0g
- Sugar: 11g

Tips:

- For a soothing effect, drink this beverage in the morning or before bed.
- If you need extra hydration, add more water to suit your taste.

8. Blueberry Yogurt Smoothie

Preparation Time:
- 10 minutes
- Serves: 4

Ingredients:
- 1 cup fresh or frozen blueberries
- 1 cup plain Greek yogurt (unsweetened)
- 1/2 cup unsweetened almond milk
- 1 tablespoon chia seeds (optional)
- 1 teaspoon vanilla extract

Instructions:
1. Blend blueberries, Greek yogurt, almond milk, chia seeds, and vanilla until smooth.
2. Adjust consistency by adding more almond milk if needed.
3. Serve chilled.

Nutritional Value (per serving):
- Calories: 110
- Carbohydrates: 18g
- Protein: 6g
- Fat: 3g
- Fiber: 4g
- Sugar: 12g

Tips:
- If you prefer a thicker smoothie, add more yogurt or frozen fruit.
- Opt for unsweetened yogurt to avoid extra sugars.

9. Avocado & Peach Smoothie

Preparation Time:
- 10 minutes
- Serves: 4

Ingredients:
- 1 ripe avocado
- 2 peaches, peeled and pitted
- 1/2 cup unsweetened almond milk
- 1 tablespoon honey (optional)
- 1/2 teaspoon cinnamon

Instructions:
1. Blend the avocado, peaches, almond milk, honey, and cinnamon until smooth.
2. If the smoothie is too thick, add more almond milk to reach the desired consistency.
3. Serve immediately.

Nutritional Value (per serving):
- Calories: 140
- Carbohydrates: 22g
- Protein: 2g
- Fat: 7g
- Fiber: 5g
- Sugar: 15g

Tips:
- The avocado adds creaminess and healthy fats to the smoothie.
- For an extra nutritional boost, add a tablespoon of flaxseeds or chia seeds.

10. Cantaloupe & Lime Slush

Preparation Time:
- 5 minutes
- Serves: 4

Ingredients:
- 3 cups cantaloupe, cubed
- 1 tablespoon lime juice
- 1/2 cup ice cubes
- 1 tablespoon honey (optional)

Instructions:
1. Blend the cantaloupe, lime juice, and ice cubes until smooth and slushy.
2. Taste and adjust sweetness with honey if desired.
3. Pour into glasses and serve chilled.

Nutritional Value (per serving):
- Calories: 60
- Carbohydrates: 16g
- Protein: 1g
- Fat: 0g
- Fiber: 2g
- Sugar: 14g

Tips:
- Use chilled cantaloupe to make the slush extra refreshing.
- You can freeze the cantaloupe cubes ahead of time for an even frostier texture.

Chapter 8

wholesome Desserts

In this chapter, you'll find desserts designed to be kind to sensitive stomachs while still fulfilling your craving for something sweet. Each recipe is made with nourishing ingredients that offer a perfect blend of flavor and comfort, using gentle, non-irritating foods. Whether you prefer baked treats, fruit-inspired desserts, or creamy indulgences, these wholesome options are meant to be both soothing and delicious, without sacrificing taste. Ideal for those looking for a more thoughtful approach to enjoying desserts.

1. Coconut Rice Pudding

Preparation Time:
- 20 minutes
- Cooking Time: 45 minutes
- Total Time: 1 hour 5 minutes
- Servings: 6

Ingredients:
- 1 cup white rice
- 2 cups coconut milk (unsweetened)
- 2 cups water
- 1/4 cup honey or maple syrup
- 1 tsp vanilla extract
- 1/4 tsp ground cinnamon (optional)
- Pinch of salt
- 1/2 cup shredded unsweetened coconut (optional)

Instructions:

1. Rinse the rice under cold water until the water runs clear.
2. In a medium saucepan, combine rice, coconut milk, water, and a pinch of salt.
3. Bring to a boil, then reduce heat to low, cover, and simmer for 40-45 minutes, or until the rice is tender and the liquid is absorbed. Stir occasionally.
4. Once cooked, stir in honey, vanilla extract, and cinnamon (if using).
5. Let cool slightly before serving. Optionally, top with shredded coconut for extra flavor.

Nutritional Value (per serving):
- Calories: 220
- Carbs: 34g
- Protein: 2g
- Fat: 10g
- Fiber: 2g
- Sugar: 12g

Tips:
- Make sure to use unsweetened coconut milk to avoid excess sugars.
- You can adjust the sweetness by adding more honey or maple syrup as desired.

2. Vanilla Almond Cake

Preparation Time:
- 15 minutes
- Baking Time: 30 minutes
- Total Time: 45 minutes
- Servings: 6

Ingredients:
- 1 1/2 cups almond flour
- 1/2 cup coconut flour
- 1 tsp baking soda
- 1/2 tsp salt
- 1/4 cup maple syrup
- 3 large eggs
- 1/4 cup coconut oil (melted)
- 1 tbsp vanilla extract

- 1/2 cup almond milk (unsweetened)

Instructions:

1. Preheat the oven to 350°F (175°C) and grease an 8-inch round cake pan.
2. In a large bowl, combine almond flour, coconut flour, baking soda, and salt.
3. In a separate bowl, whisk eggs, maple syrup, melted coconut oil, vanilla extract, and almond milk until smooth.
4. Add the wet ingredients to the dry ingredients and mix until combined.
5. Pour the batter into the prepared cake pan and bake for 30 minutes, or until a toothpick inserted comes out clean.
6. Let cool before serving.

Nutritional Value (per serving):

- Calories: 210
- Carbs: 10g
- Protein: 6g
- Fat: 18g
- Fiber: 4g

- Sugar: 5g

Tips:
- You can top the cake with a simple glaze made from powdered erythritol or a light dusting of powdered coconut.
- Almond flour is the key ingredient here, so do not substitute with other flours.

3. Blueberry Sorbet

Preparation Time:
- 10 minutes
- Freezing Time: 4 hours
- Total Time: 4 hours 10 minutes
- Servings: 6

Ingredients:
- 2 cups fresh blueberries (or frozen)
- 1/4 cup honey or maple syrup
- 1/2 cup water
- 1 tbsp lemon juice (optional)

Instructions:

1. Blend the blueberries, honey or maple syrup, water, and lemon juice (if using) in a blender until smooth.
2. Pour the mixture into a shallow pan and freeze for at least 4 hours or until solid.
3. Scrape with a fork every hour to create a light, fluffy texture.
4. Serve once the sorbet has reached a smooth consistency.

Nutritional Value (per serving):

- Calories: 100
- Carbs: 26g
- Protein: 1g
- Fat: 0g
- Fiber: 4g
- Sugar: 20g

Tips:
- If you prefer a creamier texture, you can mix in a tablespoon of coconut milk or almond milk before freezing.
- Adjust the sweetness with more or less honey depending on the sweetness of your blueberries.

4. Banana Ice Cream

Preparation Time:
- 5 minutes
- Freezing Time: 4 hours
- Total Time: 4 hours 5 minutes
- Servings: 6

Ingredients:
- 3 ripe bananas
- 1/4 cup almond milk (unsweetened)
- 1/2 tsp vanilla extract (optional)
- 1 tbsp honey (optional)

Instructions:

1. Peel and slice the bananas, then freeze the slices for at least 4 hours.
2. Blend the frozen banana slices with almond milk, vanilla extract, and honey until smooth.
3. Scoop into bowls and serve immediately for a soft-serve texture, or freeze for 30 minutes for a firmer consistency.

Nutritional Value (per serving):

- Calories: 90
- Carbs: 23g
- Protein: 1g
- Fat: 0g
- Fiber: 2g
- Sugar: 16g

Tips:

- You can experiment with adding small amounts of other fruits like strawberries or mangoes for variety.
- Serve immediately for a soft-serve texture or freeze for a firmer result.

5. Lemon Curd Cups

Preparation Time:
- 15 minutes
- Chill Time: 2 hours
- Total Time: 2 hours 15 minutes
- Servings: 6

Ingredients:
- 1/4 cup fresh lemon juice
- 1/4 cup honey or maple syrup
- 3 large eggs
- 1/4 cup butter (unsalted)
- 1 tsp vanilla extract
- 6 small gluten-free tart shells (optional)

Instructions:
1. In a medium saucepan, whisk together lemon juice, honey, and eggs.
2. Place the saucepan over low heat and cook, stirring constantly, until thickened (about 8-10 minutes).

3. Remove from heat and stir in butter and vanilla extract until smooth.

4. Let the lemon curd cool for 10 minutes, then spoon into tart shells or small cups.

5. Refrigerate for at least 2 hours before serving.

Nutritional Value (per serving):
- Calories: 180
- Carbs: 22g
- Protein: 4g
- Fat: 8g
- Fiber: 1g
- Sugar: 16g

Tips:
- If you want a richer flavor, try adding a touch of coconut cream instead of butter.
- For a smoother curd, strain it before adding to the tart shells.

6. Chocolate Avocado Mousse

Preparation Time:
- 10 minutes
- Serves: 3

Ingredients:
- 1 ripe avocado
- 3 tbsp unsweetened cocoa powder
- 2 tbsp maple syrup (or honey)
- 1 tsp vanilla extract
- 1/4 cup almond milk (or any non-dairy milk)
- Pinch of sea salt
- Fresh berries (optional, for garnish)

Instructions:
1. In a blender or food processor, combine the avocado, cocoa powder, maple syrup, vanilla extract, and almond milk.
2. Blend until smooth and creamy, scraping down the sides as needed.

3. Taste and adjust sweetness or cocoa powder as desired.

4. Spoon into serving dishes and refrigerate for at least 30 minutes to chill.

5. Top with fresh berries or a sprinkle of cocoa powder before serving.

Nutritional Value (per serving):
- Calories: 170
- Fat: 14g
- Carbs: 18g
- Fiber: 7g
- Protein: 2g

Tips:
- Use ripe avocados for the best texture and flavor.
- You can also add a pinch of cinnamon for a warm undertone without triggering sensitivities.
- For extra creaminess, add a tablespoon of coconut cream.

7. Pear & Cinnamon Crisp

Preparation Time:
- 15 minutes
- Serves: 3

Ingredients:
- 3 ripe pears, peeled and sliced
- 1/4 cup oats
- 2 tbsp almond flour
- 2 tbsp maple syrup
- 1/2 tsp ground cinnamon
- 2 tbsp coconut oil (melted)
- Pinch of sea salt

Instructions:
1. Preheat your oven to 350°F (175°C).
2. In a baking dish, arrange the pear slices evenly.
3. In a small bowl, mix the oats, almond flour, cinnamon, coconut oil, maple syrup, and sea salt until combined.
4. Sprinkle the oat mixture over the pears, covering them evenly.

5. Bake for 25-30 minutes, or until the topping is golden brown and the pears are soft.
6. Let it cool slightly before serving.

Nutritional Value (per serving):
- Calories: 220
- Fat: 11g
- Carbs: 31g
- Fiber: 6g
- Protein: 3g

Tips:

- If you prefer a sweeter dessert, drizzle a little extra maple syrup on top before serving.
- For a nutty flavor, add some chopped almonds or walnuts to the topping mixture.

8. Baked Apple with Almond Butter

Preparation Time:
- 10 minutes
- Serves: 3

Ingredients:
- 3 apples (such as Fuji or Gala)
- 3 tbsp almond butter
- 1 tsp ground cinnamon
- 1 tbsp maple syrup (optional)
- A handful of slivered almonds (optional)

Instructions:
1. Preheat your oven to 350°F (175°C).
2. Core the apples, creating a small well in the center.
3. Stuff each apple with a tablespoon of almond butter.
4. Sprinkle the apples with cinnamon, then place them in a baking dish.

5. Cover the dish with foil and bake for 20-25 minutes, or until the apples are tender.

6. Drizzle with maple syrup and sprinkle with slivered almonds before serving.

Nutritional Value (per serving):
- Calories: 190
- Fat: 14g
- Carbs: 22g
- Fiber: 5g
- Protein: 4g

Tips:
- Make sure to pick apples that hold their shape when baked.
- You can add a little bit of vanilla extract to the almond butter filling for extra flavor.

9. Carrot Cake

Preparation Time:
- 20 minutes
- Serves: 6

Ingredients:
- 1 1/2 cups grated carrots (about 3 medium carrots)
- 1/2 cup almond flour
- 1/2 cup oat flour
- 1/4 tsp baking soda
- 1/4 tsp baking powder
- 1/2 tsp ground cinnamon
- 1/4 tsp ground ginger
- 2 eggs
- 2 tbsp maple syrup
- 1/4 cup coconut oil (melted)
- 1/2 tsp vanilla extract

Instructions:

1. Preheat your oven to 350°F (175°C) and grease a small cake pan.
2. In a large bowl, whisk together the almond flour, oat flour, baking soda, baking powder, cinnamon, and ginger.
3. In another bowl, whisk the eggs, maple syrup, coconut oil, and vanilla extract.
4. Add the wet ingredients to the dry ingredients and mix until just combined.
5. Stir in the grated carrots.
6. Pour the batter into the prepared cake pan and bake for 25-30 minutes, or until a toothpick inserted comes out clean.
7. Let the cake cool before serving.

Nutritional Value (per serving):

- Calories: 220
- Fat: 16g
- Carbs: 18g
- Fiber: 4g
- Protein: 6g

Tips:
- If desired, top with a light coconut yogurt or a dairy-free frosting.
- Add a few chopped walnuts or raisins for extra texture and flavor.

10. Chia Pudding with Berries

Preparation Time:
- 5 minutes (plus overnight chilling)
- Serves: 3

Ingredients:
- 1/4 cup chia seeds
- 1 cup almond milk (or any non-dairy milk)
- 1 tbsp maple syrup (optional)
- 1/2 tsp vanilla extract
- 1/2 cup mixed berries (blueberries, raspberries, etc.)

Instructions:

1. In a bowl, combine chia seeds, almond milk, maple syrup (if using), and vanilla extract.
2. Stir well and let sit for 5 minutes.
3. Stir again, cover, and refrigerate overnight or for at least 4 hours to thicken.
4. Once set, top with fresh berries before serving.

Nutritional Value (per serving):

- Calories: 160
- Fat: 9g
- Carbs: 17g
- Fiber: 10g
- Protein: 5g

Tips:

- For a sweeter taste, add a small amount of honey or stevia to the mixture.
- You can mix in a tablespoon of almond butter for added creaminess.

Chapter 9

Meal Planning & Prep Tips

Planning your meals with Interstitial Cystitis (IC) in mind requires careful thought, as certain foods can aggravate symptoms. A well-balanced, nutrient-rich, and gentle meal plan can support overall health while minimizing flare-ups.

Step 1: Understand the Key Principles of an IC Diet

Avoid Irritants: Certain foods may trigger IC symptoms, such as acidic fruits, spicy foods, caffeine, artificial sweeteners, and alcohol.

Incorporate Soothing Foods: Emphasize anti-inflammatory, non-irritating foods like oats, bananas, leafy greens, carrots, chicken, and fish.

Balanced Nutrition: Include a mix of protein, healthy fats, fiber, and carbohydrates. This helps with overall health while ensuring you don't feel deprived.

How to Plan Your IC-Friendly 30-Day Meal Plan

Day 1-7: Starting Off Smooth & Light
Breakfast:
- Oatmeal with Blueberries & Almond Milk
- Quinoa Breakfast Bowl with Banana & Chia Seeds
- Whole Wheat Pancakes with Maple Syrup
- Scrambled Eggs with Spinach & Mushrooms
- Coconut Yogurt Parfait with Strawberries
- Avocado Toast on Gluten-Free Bread

- Rice Pudding with Cinnamon & Honey

Lunch & Dinner (Nutritious Salads & Light Meals):
- Spinach & Chicken Salad with Olive Oil Vinaigrette
- Grilled Salmon Salad with Avocado
- Carrot & Cucumber Ribbon Salad
- Roasted Beetroot Salad with Arugula
- Quinoa & Veggie Power Salad
- Chopped Cabbage Salad with Lemon Dressing
- Turkey & Cranberry Spinach Salad

Hearty Soups & Stews:
- Creamy Carrot & Ginger Soup
- Chicken & Vegetable Broth
- Butternut Squash Soup with Coconut Milk
- Potato Leek Soup
- Lentil & Spinach Stew
- Sweet Potato & Red Lentil Soup
- Tomato Basil Soup

Sides & Vegetables:
- Roasted Sweet Potato & Kale Salad
- Avocado & Tomato Salad
- Zucchini Noodles with Lemon
- Roasted Garlic & Herb Sweet Potatoes
- Steamed Asparagus with Lemon Zest
- Sautéed Spinach with Olive Oil & Garlic
- Baked Zucchini Fries

Healthy Snacks & Treats:
- Carrot & Cucumber Sticks with Hummus
- Grilled Veggie Skewers
- Apple Slices with Peanut Butter
- Rice Cakes with Avocado Spread
- Cucumber & Cream Cheese Bites
- Carrot Sticks with Tzatziki
- Baked Zucchini Chips

Smoothies & Refreshing Beverages:
- Green Smoothie with Spinach & Banana
- Berry Almond Milk Smoothie
- Tropical Mango Coconut Smoothie
- Cucumber & Mint Infused Water
- Sweet Carrot & Apple Juice
- Pear & Ginger Smoothie
- Lemon & Honey Detox Drink

Dessert:
- Coconut Rice Pudding
- Vanilla Almond Cake
- Blueberry Sorbet
- Banana Ice Cream
- Lemon Curd Cups
- Chocolate Avocado Mousse
- Pear & Cinnamon Crisp

Day 8-14: Exploring More Hearty Options

Breakfast:
- Sweet Potato Hash
- Apple Cinnamon Quinoa
- Scrambled Eggs with Spinach & Mushrooms
- Oatmeal with Blueberries & Almond Milk
- Banana Nut Smoothie
- Quinoa Breakfast Bowl with Banana & Chia Seeds
- Whole Wheat Pancakes with Maple Syrup

Lunch & Dinner (Nutritious Salads & Light Meals):
- Roasted Sweet Potato & Kale Salad
- Avocado & Tomato Salad
- Grilled Salmon Salad with Avocado
- Turkey & Cranberry Spinach Salad
- Spinach & Chicken Salad with Olive Oil Vinaigrette

- Chopped Cabbage Salad with Lemon Dressing
- Roasted Beetroot Salad with Arugula

Hearty Soups & Stews:
- Beef & Root Vegetable Stew
- Chicken Bone Broth with Carrots
- Broccoli & Cauliflower Cream Soup
- Butternut Squash Soup with Coconut Milk
- Potato Leek Soup
- Tomato Basil Soup
- Sweet Potato & Red Lentil Soup

Sides & Vegetables:
- Quinoa & Vegetable Stir-Fry
- Roasted Garlic & Herb Sweet Potatoes
- Steamed Asparagus with Lemon Zest
- Sautéed Spinach with Olive Oil & Garlic
- Cauliflower Rice Pilaf
- Mashed Butternut Squash
- Roasted Brussels Sprouts with Apple Cider Vinegar

Healthy Snacks & Treats:
- Carrot & Cucumber Sticks with Hummus
- Grilled Veggie Skewers
- Apple Slices with Peanut Butter
- Rice Cakes with Avocado Spread
- Cucumber & Cream Cheese Bites
- Carrot Sticks with Tzatziki
- Baked Zucchini Chips

Smoothies & Refreshing Beverages:
- Pear & Ginger Smoothie
- Lemon & Honey Detox Drink
- Blueberry Yogurt Smoothie
- Avocado & Peach Smoothie
- Cantaloupe & Lime Slush
- Coconut Rice Pudding

Tropical Mango Coconut Smoothie Dessert:
- Chocolate Avocado Mousse
- Banana Ice Cream

- Pear & Cinnamon Crisp
- Carrot Cake
- Chia Pudding with Berries
- Baked Apple with Almond Butter
- Coconut Macaroons with Fruit Popsicles

Day 15-21: Mid-Month & Meal Variations

Breakfast:
- Scrambled Eggs with Spinach & Mushrooms
- Avocado Toast on Gluten-Free Bread
- Oatmeal with Blueberries & Almond Milk
- Banana Nut Smoothie
- Sweet Potato Hash
- Quinoa Breakfast Bowl with Banana & Chia Seeds
- Rice Pudding with Cinnamon & Honey
- Lunch & Dinner (Nutritious Salads & Light Meals):
- Grilled Cod with Sweet Potato Mash

- Zucchini Noodles with Chicken & Olive Oil
- Eggplant Parmesan
- Roasted Chicken with Green Beans
- Veggie-Stuffed Bell Peppers
- Turkey Meatballs with Quinoa
- Baked Salmon with Steamed Veggies

Hearty Soups & Stews:
- Lentil & Spinach Stew
- Broccoli & Cauliflower Cream Soup
- Chicken & Vegetable Broth
- Butternut Squash Soup with Coconut Milk
- Sweet Potato & Red Lentil Soup
- Beef & Root Vegetable Stew
- Tomato Basil Soup

Sides & Vegetables:
- Roasted Garlic & Herb Sweet Potatoes
- Steamed Asparagus with Lemon Zest
- Sautéed Spinach with Olive Oil & Garlic
- Baked Zucchini Fries

- Cauliflower Rice Pilaf
- Mashed Butternut Squash
- Roasted Brussels Sprouts with Apple Cider Vinegar

Healthy Snacks & Treats:
- Apple Slices with Peanut Butter
- Rice Cakes with Avocado Spread
- Cucumber & Cream Cheese Bites
- Carrot Sticks with Tzatziki
- Baked Zucchini Chips
- Homemade Popcorn with Olive Oil
- Frozen Yogurt Bark with Berries

Smoothies & Refreshing Beverages:
- Blueberry Yogurt Smoothie
- Green Smoothie with Spinach & Banana
- Tropical Mango Coconut Smoothie
- Cucumber & Mint Infused Water
- Sweet Carrot & Apple Juice
- Pear & Ginger Smoothie
- Lemon & Honey Detox Drink

Dessert:
- Chia Pudding with Berries
- Vanilla Almond Cake
- Blueberry Sorbet
- Banana Ice Cream
- Lemon Curd Cups
- Chocolate Avocado Mousse
- Pear & Cinnamon Crisp

Day 22-30: Wrapping Up the Month with Comfort & Creativity

Breakfast:
- Whole Wheat Pancakes with Maple Syrup
- Avocado Toast on Gluten-Free Bread
- Rice Pudding with Cinnamon & Honey
- Oatmeal with Blueberries & Almond Milk
- Quinoa Breakfast Bowl with Banana & Chia Seeds
- Scrambled Eggs with Spinach & Mushrooms
- Banana Nut Smoothie

Lunch & Dinner (Nutritious Salads & Light Meals):
- Spinach & Chicken Salad with Olive Oil Vinaigrette
- Grilled Lemon Herb Chicken with Rice
- Baked Tilapia with Sautéed Spinach
- Grilled Salmon Salad with Avocado
- Zucchini Noodles with Chicken & Olive Oil
- Veggie-Stuffed Bell Peppers
- Roasted Sweet Potato & Kale Salad

Hearty Soups & Stews:
- Chicken & Vegetable Broth
- Butternut Squash Soup with Coconut Milk
- Beef & Root Vegetable Stew
- Potato Leek Soup
- Tomato Basil Soup
- Lentil & Spinach Stew
- Sweet Potato & Red Lentil Soup

Sides & Vegetables:
- Steamed Asparagus with Lemon Zest
- Roasted Garlic & Herb Sweet Potatoes
- Sautéed Spinach with Olive Oil & Garlic
- Cauliflower Rice Pilaf
- Mashed Butternut Squash
- Roasted Brussels Sprouts with Apple Cider Vinegar
- Grilled Veggie Skewers

Healthy Snacks & Treats:
- Almond Protein Bars
- Carrot & Cucumber Sticks with Hummus
- Rice Cakes with Avocado Spread
- Carrot Sticks with Tzatziki
- Baked Zucchini Chips
- Homemade Popcorn with Olive Oil
- Coconut Macaroons with Fruit Popsicles

Smoothies & Refreshing Beverages:
- Tropical Mango Coconut Smoothie
- Pear & Ginger Smoothie
- Green Smoothie with Spinach & Banana
- Blueberry Yogurt Smoothie
- Sweet Carrot & Apple Juice
- Cucumber & Mint Infused Water
- Lemon & Honey Detox Drink

Dessert:
- Coconut Rice Pudding
- Vanilla Almond Cake
- Chocolate Avocado Mousse
- Banana Ice Cream
- Pear & Cinnamon Crisp
- Blueberry Sorbet
- Lemon Curd Cups

By following this 30-day IC (Interstitial Cystitis) diet meal prep plan, you can tailor your meals to meet your specific dietary needs while staying within a healthy 1500-calorie goal. This plan offers a variety of delicious, easy-to-make meals that support your bladder health and avoid common irritants associated with IC. Whether you're managing symptoms, maintaining your current health, or simply seeking a balanced diet, this meal plan provides flexibility while ensuring you stay comfortable. With a little preparation, you'll have nutritious, bladder-friendly meals ready for the entire month, making it easier to stay on track with your health goals.

Batch Cooking and Freezer-Friendly Recipes

Batch cooking can save time and ensure you always have IC-friendly meals ready to go. Consider cooking large portions of soups, stews, quinoa, and roasted vegetables at once. Freeze them in portion-sized containers for easy access on busy days.

Grocery Shopping on the IC Diet

When shopping for an IC diet, stick to whole, unprocessed foods like lean meats, fish, vegetables, and gluten-free grains. Make sure to avoid foods like tomatoes, citrus fruits, caffeine, and alcohol.

Best Pantry Staples for IC Diet Success

Grains: Quinoa, brown rice, oats, and gluten-free pasta.
Proteins: Chicken, turkey, fish, and tofu.

Fruits & Vegetables: Spinach, zucchini, carrots, sweet potatoes, and bananas.

Dairy Alternatives: Almond milk, coconut yogurt.

Healthy Fats: Olive oil, avocado, and almond butter.

With these tips and meal options, you're ready to embark on a month of nourishing, IC-friendly meals!

Conclusion

To conclude, the Super Easy IC Diet Cookbook is an essential resource for those dealing with Interstitial Cystitis (IC), providing simple and practical recipes tailored to the specific dietary needs of IC sufferers. By following the suggested dietary guidelines, readers can reduce symptoms, improve bladder function, and promote overall well-being.

Final Thoughts on Maintaining Long-Term Bladder Health

Maintaining long-term bladder health is an ongoing process that involves consistent effort, mindful food choices, and making necessary lifestyle adjustments. Adopting an IC-friendly diet can help alleviate flare-ups, support healing, and sustain healthy bladder function. Staying informed and proactive about what you eat plays a crucial role in improving your quality of life.

Monitoring Your Progress

Tracking your progress is a vital part of managing IC effectively. By recording your meals, symptoms, and any changes, you can pinpoint which foods are beneficial or problematic for your condition. Keeping a journal or using an app to track these factors allows you to make informed decisions, adjust your diet as needed, and work closely with your healthcare team to achieve the best results.

Support and Community Resources for IC

Finally, finding support and engaging with others who are living with IC can make a big difference. Many online communities, forums, and organizations offer valuable resources, advice, and emotional support for individuals coping with IC. Connecting with others can provide a sense of belonging, shared experiences, and encouragement in your journey to manage your condition effectively.

Made in the USA
Las Vegas, NV
23 March 2025